Everything You Never Learned about Sex

Take Back Your Masculine Power & Use Your Sex Energy for Good

Everything You Never Learned about Sex

Take Back Your Masculine Power & Use Your Sex Energy for Good

Michael McPherson

CHANGEMAKERS
BOOKS

Winchester, UK
Washington, USA

JOHN HUNT PUBLISHING

First published by Changemakers Books, 2021
Changemakers Books is an imprint of John Hunt Publishing Ltd., No. 3 East Street,
Alresford, Hampshire SO24 9EE, UK
office@jhpbooks.com
www.johnhuntpublishing.com
www.changemakers-books.com

For distributor details and how to order please visit the 'Ordering' section on our website.

ISBN: 978 1 78904 638 0
978 1 78904 639 7 (ebook)
Library of Congress Control Number: 2020938312

A CIP catalogue record for this book is available from the British Library.

Design: Stuart Davies

UK: Printed and bound by CPI Group (UK) Ltd, Croydon, CR0 4YY
Printed in North America by CPI GPS partners

Contents

For my daughter, my yet to be born baby girl, Daddy loves you.

For my wife, may the ripple effect of this work echo your effect on me. I love you.

During times of universal deceit, telling the truth becomes a revolutionary act.
George Orwell

Introduction

I'm not your standard expert on sex. In a world where credentials and intellectual knowledge often weigh in above vulnerability, authenticity, heart-centered expression, and embodiment, I hope this book, and me as the author of it, inspires you to look within yourself and discover your own inner expert. I take full responsibility for the man I am. I don't pretend to be a guru or an enlightened master of any kind. I was born the same way you were, innocently human. In my adolescent years, I was oddly troubled by the world. The repression that pervaded my immediate environment impacted me deeply. I grew up feeling different from those I loved. Instead of celebrating my differences, I shunned them, wanting so badly to feel some sense of belonging. I repressed myself, and because I did, my relationship to sex was molded by misinformation and fear. Nearly twenty years later, I've finally popped out the other side. I've stepped out of the fear-based paradigm and embraced a more loving relationship with sex. I'm here to help you do the same. Healing my relationship with sex and the opposite sex didn't come without its challenges. You'll be challenged too. It's an uphill climb, but gratefully, we have all the tools we need to succeed.

I dream of a day when our collective sex energy is utilized as our greatest catalyst for creating unconditional love in the world, a day when we embrace our inherent innocence and see that innocence when we look at each other. I dream of a day when we open our hearts to the true transcendental power of sex; two becoming one and creating a third, a love-based awareness that will become the future consciousness of this planet. Let's face it, the world needs that kind of love right now. As I write this, humanity faces one of its gravest challenges yet, the revival of the human heart. Across our globe we are seeing entire ecosystems in collapse, mass extinctions of flora and fauna, unprecedented environmental pollution, human driven climate change, and a complete over exhaustion of the Earth's natural resources. That's only what we're doing to the Earth. Our crimes against each other include war, genocide, extreme poverty, denied access to basic human needs, healthcare systems that neither care nor have anything to do with health, poisoned foods, water, air, skincare products, and medications, government officials serving corporate interests, military privatization, voter fraud and political lobbying, corporate greed undermining democracy, fractional reserve banking and unrestrained inflation, and a near monopoly of the world's resources, all while mainstream media distracts us from the very real issues of our time under the guise of "entertainment." Sounds grim, I know, but whether you believe it or not, we're all in the middle of a global crisis. Given her multi-billion year existence, it's not the Earth's future that's in question. It's our own.

I'm often asked, "what's the point?" As in, why do all this work to embody such love in love-making? Why not just surrender into our ever-obvious "animalistic" nature? Sex is a melting pot for both the best and the worst in humanity. If we can heal the greed, selfishness, objectivity, corruption, immaturity, and superficiality latent in our sexuality, then we can heal those same things in our world. If we can restore the full power of the human heart into our relationship with sex, then we can elicit the most powerful creative force in the universe to go to work on manifesting the real, effective, and lasting heart-centered solutions for our current global crisis. We can consciously unleash our sacred sexual life force and use it to begin reconstructing our world on the basis of love instead of fear. We have beneath our belts the power to create entirely new realities, but only those creations joined with love will lift humanity out of its current crisis and into the higher harmonies of the heart.

It takes a truly courageous individual to lean into those dark, uncomfortable, and unexplored spaces within themselves and be with them until they reveal their wisdom. I honor you for your bravery, for your willingness to step into the unknown, to feel both your pain and your inherent innocence. I eagerly anticipate the goodness that is to come as a result of your work. Intimacy and connection have always been an essential part of what it means to be human, but in many ways, we're only now recognizing our capacity for co-creating such experiences. Sex has long been a taboo subject, something that we as a collective have intentionally bypassed out of our fear of feeling it all, both the ecstatic highs of heart-orgasming bliss and the despairing lows of our devastating present and past. Healing the wounds of our ancestry is not for the faint of heart, especially when it comes to a topic as sensitive as this. Healing, however, is what we're here to do, and now is the time that we embrace our mission whole-heartedly.

Over the course of history, it's most often been the men of society that have perpetuated the misuse of sex, using it to attain power and suppress the feminine body and all that it represents. This is one of the main reasons we have such resistance to leaning into this conversation. We know we've contributed to the misuse of sex. Personally, I've been the manipulator, the womanizer, the one objectifying, and the man that only approached sex from the perspective of what he could get out of it. In being all those things, I've lived on both sides of the battle. I've been lost in darkness and found my way back to the light. I've left a long trail of broken relationships, broken hearts, and pain in my wake, contributing to my fair share of the wounding between the sexes, but I intend to make it right.

This whole book is a massive invitation for the men of my generation to assume radical responsibility for the wounds of our personal and collective past. It goes without saying that uncomfortable things will come up. If they don't, then you're not reading it right. In other words, you're not allowing this message to really hit you. I invite you to do just that. I invite you to allow this message to penetrate you on a cellular level, so that together, we can begin carving out a new, inspired, and aligned expression of our sexuality. Not only for us, but for every generation that will walk in our footsteps. They are looking to us now as the role models for what it means to be a man. It's up to us to show them that being a man very much means living with an open heart, both inside and outside of the bedroom.

In this book, I'll share with you aspects of my story that you will relate to. If I do my job, then I'll effectively mirror back to you an aspect of yourself that's desiring to be healed, upgraded, and returned to love. It's your job to do that work. I know you will because I know you're ready. You wouldn't be holding this book in your hands if you weren't. I also know there's a generation of women out there longing for the return of the sacred masculine, longing for the men that will once again honor sex and the female body as sacred. We shall not disappoint. The good news is, everything we need to accomplish our mission, to restore the heart into human sexuality, already exists within us. We needn't look any further than our physical body and the wisdom that dwells inside. You've been divinely equipped for this journey. It's one that you signed up for long before you were born. Trust in that knowing.

Arriving on the heels of the "me too" movement this book and the message within it seems more relevant than ever. If we as men cannot learn to properly channel our sexual energy for the greatest good, how can we ever expect to protect our boys and girls from sexual violence, let alone teach them about the wonders of sex, intimacy, relationship, and pleasure? It's clear now, there is a problem, and no one movement, organization, or educational platform will be the answer. This is a fundamentally human issue and its implications reach down to the very core of what it means to be human. It's equal rights for all people regardless of our apparent differences, and it starts in the heart of each person willing to take radical responsibility for their part, whatever that part may be. This is a time of healing. It would be negligent for any of us to believe that we don't have a unique role to play in that healing, just as we've had in the creation of the suffering.

Throughout this book I'll give voice to some of my personal experiences regarding my sexual upbringing, including how these experiences influenced my reality and how that reality impacted my life and the lives of those that came into relationship with me. I'll share with you the lessons I've learned along the way. This book is a healthy mix of my own personal narrative and a presentation of what my life experiences have invited me to learn and embody. We'll look at the big picture context like our modern patriarchal system and how it influences and drives our culture, as well as the more individual context of what you can do to begin reshaping your personal relationship with sex.

My intention with this work is to encourage the evolution of a new species of man, one that's shamelessly connected to his sexual power and channeling that power in service to the love in his heart. Included in this vision is a man that understands and honors the feminine, upholds the integrity of his divinely appointed creative life force, approaches sex with reverence and respect, and stands tall in protecting all that is sacred. Together we're journeying back to our innocence, the "we" we were (and still are) before any of our adopted conditionings. All of this will strengthen our ability to use our sex energy for good.

I'm not here to fix or change you in any way. I don't believe you're broken. In fact, it's because of who you are that I was inspired to write this book. I've seen such goodness in the hearts of men. My job is simple, remind you of all that you already are and encourage you to see that within yourself. The fear and shame that has kept us small and divided has had its time. We can appreciate the contrast for what it taught us, while at the same time choosing to release the lower frequencies of sex once and for all.

This doesn't mean we'll be perfect by any means. You have to understand that we've been conditioned our entire lives to view sex and our sexuality through a certain lens. We didn't wind up being who we are today overnight. Therefore, we shouldn't expect to undo a lifetime of conditioning all in one day. This transition takes time, commitment, focus, courage, and a willingness to feel the full depth of emotion that's been warehoused in our body. Our mind often understands what happened as well as what we made it mean long before our body feels ready to acknowledge the hurt and let it go. This is the practice of embodiment, to take what we know to be true in our mind and have that truth resonate in our body.

Give it time. Have patience for your process and compassion for the ways you've been conditioned since you were a child. The thoughts you think that make you believe you're a bad person and the shame you still carry around your sexuality, were never yours to begin with. They were borrowed from a previous generation, programmed into you to keep you small. It's not your fault you absorbed them like a sponge. If you're willing to be responsible for them, they can end here with us, without needing to be passed on to our children.

Ultimately, honoring sex as sacred and restoring the heart back into our human sexuality is our gift to ourselves. There is so much to receive in honoring sex and our creative life force as sacred. We are the real beneficiaries of this work. Receiving is the spiritual work of the twenty-first century (which I'll cover towards the end of this book). Fully receiving the gift of love-making brings us right up against our deepest sense of unworthiness. How could we be worthy of such love? We, the imperfect person with all the mistakes we've made; how could we be worthy of such unconditional love? Well, my friends, that I leave up to you to discover; the discovery of which is everything you've been looking for.

Last item of importance here. Take what feels right to you and leave the rest. In no way am I pretending to be the be-all and end-all for the topic of sex. These teachings are what have made themselves known to me through my life experiences. In that sense, they're unique to me. Be as open as possible to contemplating them, receiving them, and applying them to your life. I won't be offended if something doesn't resonate. Each of us is on our own unique journey. What resonates as truth for you will be unique to wherever you are on your journey. Remember, you're the ultimate source of truth and wisdom for your life. Ideally, this material will only ever lead you home to yourself, your inner-truths, and the source of wisdom that lives in you. If at any point it gets confusing, or something doesn't quite feel right to you, close your eyes and place your hands over your heart. Take a few deep breaths and ask yourself, "what is it that's trying to reveal itself to me right now?" Listen for the answer. Trust what you hear. I promise your heart will never mislead you.

Chapter 1

The Best Story Never Told

I feel like every man must remember his first time masturbating. After all, it is a pivotal turning point in every man's life, at least it was for me. It was like one day, out of nowhere and for no reason at all, I felt the sudden urge to explore myself. Sitting there on my parents' toilet in the hallway bathroom (sorry mom and dad), curiosity overcame me. As if I had instinctively known how to do this all along, I began massaging myself in a way that inspired arousal. Looking back, I obviously had no idea what I was doing, but on that day, something ancient had awoken in me, switching on my impulse to explore. Stroke after stroke this instinctual impulse grew. I remember thinking, "wow, this actually feels really good. Oh my God, what is that feeling? Oh... oh... oh... holy shit!" That ten seconds of orgasmic bliss was something I would easily spend the next fifteen years of my life chasing.

That moment, that pure, potent, pristine moment of experiencing my sex energy for the first time and feeling the fundamental creative life force that inhabits my body, was truly magical... and completely innocent. I was blown away by the whole experience, in shock actually. I had no idea my body was capable of feeling such pleasure. Never before had I felt anything like it. All my innocent and enthusiastic mind could think of at the time was, "whoa, I want to do that again." So, naturally, I did. Little did I know that in those moments, I was initiating my post-pubescent transition into manhood. This incident, albeit brief, was easily the most spectacular discovery I had ever made. Immediately inspired to learn everything I could about what it was I had just experienced, my mind raced with both the excitement and fear I felt around the whole situation. "Had my friends known about this? Had they known all along? If so, why hadn't they said anything? Maybe I shouldn't either… I don't want to seem like a newbie." One thing was clear, I had just discovered magic! But who could I talk to about this?

Turns out that sex isn't a topic spoken about openly amongst most Midwestern American families, especially those in the religious sector. Outside of a few sessions of Sex Ed during my sixth-grade science class, when officer Eddie, a big, burly, gargantuan of a man, would come in and share about the horrors of sex, sexually transmitted diseases, and teenage pregnancy, intentionally doing his best to scare the hell out of us… nothing. Personal note here, kids should never have to see the slide show horrors that we had to witness at such a young age. Like whoa, pump the brakes there good God-fearing Catholics. Believe me, this is awkward for all of us. We were just kids wanting to do kid things. I was far more interested in the pet iguana my science teacher kept in our sixth-grade classroom than I ever was in the pet iguana in my pants, let alone what I could do with it.

Really though, nothing. No father-son convos, no getting together with buddies and one by one sharing our sexual experiences, no cartoons, TV shows, classes, books, or mentors to walk us through the ever-obvious hormonal changes happening in our body. Just pictures of herpes, that's what we got. So, rather than facing my fears of what my parents might say, what the doctor might say, what my educators might say, and what my friends might say, I did what any teenage boy does when faced with something emotionally challenging, I internalized it. I quickly decided that my safest bet, and the one least likely to result in embarrassment, was to explore this topic further in private. No way was I going to risk speaking up about something so controversial, especially when I had little to no knowledge of it myself.

With the Internet being practically accessible to anyone and Instant Messenger being all the rage back in the early 2000s, keeping us youngsters at our family computers virtually 24/7, eagerly waiting to see who might jump on and want to chat, porn became the clearest option for exploring this new arena of sex. Other than the pretty much constant fear of getting caught, which only ever amplified the adrenaline rush, porn felt like a safe space to explore sex. There was also an element of control. No one could push me past my boundaries or make me feel embarrassed about being inexperienced. My intention with porn was only ever to get familiar enough with sex to feel some sense of confidence around it. But the porn industry obviously had other intentions for us post-pubescent boys. Whether you agree with it or not, porn is what educated me and all my friends about sex. If you know anything about porn, which I'm certain you do, then you know that its primary goal is not education, it's entertainment. As my educator, porn was spectacular at teaching me how to dehumanize human beings and sexually objectify women.

There were no laptops back then, so the family computer was the only option. I can't even begin to tell you how many times I masturbated to porn right in the middle of our family living room, my parents just on the other side of the wall either watching television or making dinner. Kind of ironic considering how much I was learning about sex from the comfort of my own home, just not from the people that I was meant to be learning from. It was like this whole new world, one that had been previously concealed from my awareness, was suddenly blasted open. Every single novelty imaginable was up for grabs. My mind was flooding with imagery that, for all I knew, was what sex was. Understanding next to nothing about the subject, I was operating with a laser-like focus in light of how much I felt I had to learn.

I quickly became addicted to the surge of dopamine and other neurochemicals that released in my brain every time I opened up that web browser and put my hand down my pants.

It started out being pretty infrequent, as I was naturally fearful of getting caught. As my confidence grew, so did the frequency of my online visits. It got to the point where I didn't even need the footage anymore to feel that drop of dopamine. All I had to do was think about watching porn, something that wasn't too terribly difficult for my mind to do, and the feel-good chemicals would start dumping in. I was like one of those Pavlovian dogs, foaming at the mouth at the sound of dinner bells, my mind and body anticipating what was to come.

Given my generation (millennials) was the first childhood generation to grow up with virtually unlimited access to Internet porn, it wasn't until much later into my adulthood that I became aware of porn's harmful effects on human brain chemistry. Scientific studies reveal that porn is one of the most addictive and damaging substances that a young, developing mind can be exposed to. It's now understood that porn consumption contributes to the underdevelopment of the prefrontal cortex, an area of the brain responsible for intellectual maturity and decision making. Add in the fact that the male brain doesn't fully develop until a man's early thirties, and you've got yourself a true developmental nightmare—one that we're only now starting to grasp.

Porn exposed my innocent mind to genres of sex that I could have never imagined on my own; things like incest, gangbanging, anal, fetishes, hardcore, MILF, and hentai. It very much warped my developing reality around sex; how to have it, how to treat a woman, what made a man a desirable sex partner, what made a woman feel pleasure, what was absolutely essential in order to reign supreme in the bedroom. As a teenager and young adult, I used to think that women only wanted to have sex with men that had huge penises and could "destroy" them in the bedroom. Being a man of average size, I quickly realized I was doomed to sexual mediocrity unless I did something about it. I'll never forget the day that I opened up to my mother about all this. Hands shaking, heart racing, voice stumbling, I asked her if there was any way to, you know, "make it bigger." She laughed that uncomfortable laugh that only a mother in her position could do under such awkward circumstances. It was enough for me to never open up about it again.

Instead, I took it upon myself to order those "magic pills" advertised on Internet porn sites. You know, the ones that promised to make you inches bigger in weeks. When those didn't work, and after having the horrible scare of my best friend finding them in the bottom drawer of my dresser (don't worry, I said they were my dad's), I graduated to what I thought might be a more sophisticated option, a penis enlargement device. And no, if you're wondering, that didn't work either. It only gave me constant anxiety that someone would catch me wearing it and my life would be over. Not to mention how ridiculously uncomfortable it was to wear. From all apparent perspectives, and after much effort on my behalf, it was clear my cards had been dealt. I would never be a Peter North or a Lexington Steele, but I would certainly make the most of what I had been given. Needless to say, I entered into the realm of sex with a boatload of insecurities, but I was ready to do whatever it would take to be a man.

As my porn consumption continued, I began adopting pornography's portrayal of women as sex objects, both on and off the screen. I unconsciously took out the "human factor." Rather than viewing women as people; loved ones, sisters, daughters, mothers, and even children themselves, I was unconsciously training my brain to view women as objects relevant for nothing more than my viewing pleasure. As a teenager, I found myself playing out these sexual fantasies with the women in my life. The more I took into my mind through the computer screen, the more the barriers diminished between this virtual reality I was observing in private and the actual reality I was living in every day. The further I progressed into adulthood, the more distracting these fantasies became, causing me to become aroused at inappropriate times and in asexual situations. It started to feel like anything I experienced my mind could twist into some kind of sexual fantasy. It didn't even feel under my control anymore.

My mind was clearly operating on a new software system it had adopted from porn. Everywhere I went I was checking girls out, looking them up and down, and almost immediately deciding whether or not I would have sex with them. I was hungry to feed my sexual appetite, but no matter how much I indulged it with pornography and masturbation, I still felt like I was starving for more. On the outside, everything seemed peachy; great grades, athletic success, captain of all my sports teams, lots of friends, and plenty of extracurriculars. Inside, I was developing a pornographic lens through which I was viewing the world, never quite realizing there were any other options to choose from.

Add alcohol into the mix, something that typically gets introduced into a man's life around the same time that his sex hormones come online, and you're starting to get a good feel for how most Western millennial men developed sexually. I started drinking when I was sixteen. Alcohol quickly became my gateway to exploring these sexual fantasies with real women. That was the whole point after all, right? Otherwise, I was only developing a profound relationship with our family computer and my dominant hand. I was way too chicken shit to pursue my sexual desires with the opposite sex sober. It was too scary for me. So, I drank, a lot, and eventually developed a functional relationship with this so called "liquid encouragement." Drinking alcohol helped most of the barriers to sexual engagement come down. It also gave me access to sex without needing to be at all developed in other things like vulnerability, authenticity, openness, and honesty.

With alcohol, I didn't even need to care. All I had to do

was show up, drink enough, and inevitably there would be someone there from the opposite sex that had done the same. Unfortunately, my many years of masturbating to pornography had inconveniently developed into a condition known as premature ejaculation, something that riddled me with anxiety any time the opportunity to have sex presented itself. Turns out that building a superficial relationship to sex that's entirely focused on the end result of ejaculation doesn't exactly help when it comes to prolonged sexual pleasure. Alcohol helped with that too. When the alcohol wasn't enough, there was always the reliable TROJAN Extended Pleasure condom that was capable of numbing pretty much everything down there. The first time I had sex I was drunk, high, and just barely conscious enough to feel anything at all. I was also in the same room as three of my closest high school buddies that were all doing the same thing. The blood on the bed sheets let me know that it was her first time too, probably the reason she started crying as soon as it was all over. Thank God her friends were there to console her, because I was far too gone to be of any good use.

As time went on, so did the sexual encounters not all that different from the one above, except now I was gaining experience. As the numbers climbed so did my sense of security around being a man. Somehow, I had gotten those things collapsed: sleeping with a lot of women and being a man. I started to relate to my sexual history as a badge of honor. Turns out my ability to seduce women was a skill highly sought after by the other guys my age. The more notches on my belt, the more I was valued as a "ladies' man," or at least that's how it felt. Women talked too and my reputation quickly got around. Oddly enough, my behavior seemed to be celebrated by both sexes.

Through guys acknowledging me as a "player" with slaps on the back and arms around the shoulders, and the women my age revering me as some kind of pre-2012 *Magic Mike*, I started to feel like more of a man for myself. I had become one of those mythological "cool kids." My badge of honor had me feeling like I finally fitted in. I had graduated into the hall of fame of manhood and my promiscuity was what had gotten me there. My manhood was totally contingent on adding more notches to my belt. Looking back, I was only ever coping with my insecurities, trying to prove myself a man, seeking validation from the women I slept with and the men that later found out about it. The only problem was, not only had I not yet learned how to face my insecurities, but my whole idea of what it meant to be a man was based on some synthetic reality I had seen online. I actually thought that being a man meant masquerading around like some kind of New Age Casanova.

Constantly seeking validation for my manliness felt like a tireless journey. No matter how often I was having sex, just below the surface, the same question always remained, "am I really a man?" My entire identity had now been constructed around being skilled with women. Sure, I played the part of being a charismatic danger to every woman in sight, but in reality, I didn't have a monstrous penis, I wasn't 6'5" and chiseled, and I would certainly never be as dominant as the men I witnessed in porn. That haunted me. So, I strived to be more like them. I did my best to embody what they modeled to me as "manly." Just beneath the surface, I still felt terrified of being with a woman, especially sober. My heart was intuitively craving intimacy and connection, but my porn programming was screaming "don't be a pussy. Man up." I was afraid of being seen as a weakling. Even more so, I was afraid of taking off the mask and spilling my vulnerabilities to someone that could turn around and weaponize them. I wasn't ready to trust anyone with that kind of ammunition. Even though I was genuinely desiring something real, fear kept me repressed. Fear kept my heart closed like a clam.

Eventually I would ease my way into romantic relationships,

but the first time I ever innocently opened up my heart to what felt like true love, I ended up heartbroken. When I did end up giving love a second chance, entering into an on and off relationship that lasted nearly five years, again I ended up heartbroken. It took me quite a while to get over that one. For years I slept around with strangers and even dated a few times secretly hoping my ex would take me back. Instead I watched her sail away with the man of her dreams while I bounced around from one relationship to the next, always one foot in and one foot out, dating half-heartedly. I had become well versed at keeping my heart closed, especially since I already knew how it was all going to go. Eventually, the relationship would end, most likely on bad terms, at which point I would blame her for "being crazy" and within days move on to the next girl. From my perspective, I was doing myself a favor by keeping my heart closed, saving myself from the inevitable heartbreak I would feel once it all came crashing down.

Bruised and calloused, guardedness, defensiveness, and reaction became my new normal. Outside of my relationships, I seemed like a delightful guy. Inside my relationships, I was creating mess after mess with no real intention of cleaning it up. Over the course of the next three romantic relationships (seven months, nine months, and just over a year), I discovered that real romance is pretty challenging. If I wanted something real, it was going to take a lot of work on my behalf. Up until that point, I had settled for blaming my partners for all of our relationship problems, never once noticing the single constant, me. At some point, right around three to six months, I would predictably breakdown, lash out in anger, and project all my past heartbreak onto my partner. I always made sure to correlate our relationship problems with her "mommy and daddy issues."

There I was, a twenty something-year-old by society's standards successful adult with everything going for him; handsome, intelligent, quick witted, physically fit. The world was my oyster, or at least that's what everyone kept telling me. Along the way I had picked up some cute little nicknames like "Mr. Perfect," "Superman," and "Captain America," because from the outside looking in, I was the perfect package. My insides revealed a very different story. I was heartbroken, hurt, emotionally stunted, and sexually immature. Outside of getting through life's basics like eating, working, exercising, and sleeping, I tended to focus all of my energy on partying, dating apps, and hooking up with strangers. All my unresolved hurt haunted me, as did my continual use of pornography and one-night stands. It felt like someone had attached a vacuum to my heart and was slowly but thoroughly sucking away my soul. I felt like a total fraud that had somehow duped everyone else into believing he was happy.

My external success masked my internal struggle. Rarely did anyone recognize how much I was suffering inside. Sprinkle in the drama of having recently divorced myself from the Catholic Church, the uproar that would cause in my family, my growing desperation to nail down a career, my massive student loan debt, and you're starting to get a real feel for the many layers of complexity that kept men like me from maturing sexually.

Where were my role models? Where were the men in my life encouraging me to cultivate a deeper relationship with myself? Where were those resourceful men when I needed them, the ones that could guide me in navigating puberty, sex, sexual desire, women, vulnerability, and channeling my creative life force? The ones that could talk me through romantic relationships, sit me down and explore with me what it meant to be a man, how to connect with my purpose? Where were the men that could show me how to handle heartbreak, give me permission to feel it, help me reopen my heart, and teach me to share it vulnerably?

I believe my story is one of the more common stories of how innocent boys become the hurt, closed hearted, emotionally underdeveloped, and sexually stunted men that populate modern society; the men that eventually pass their hurt onto others. Most of us didn't experience any of what society deems as real trauma; no sexual violence, molestation, abuse in the family household, intense poverty, loss of loved ones, freak accidents or near-death experiences. From all apparent perspectives, it looked like we had the perfect young life; loving family, good friends, great education, privileged young life experiences, and parents that provided for all of our basic needs. Why, then, was I was going through my midlife crisis at twenty-five? Was I just a "special needs" kid that had never been properly diagnosed? Or had I somehow slipped through the cracks without receiving the equipment required for a truly fulfilling life? Where had I gone wrong?

It all comes down to one simple fact: I, like all of us, was born "sensitive." Yes, that nine letter word that every man hates being associated with. With no one there to guide me through my innately sensitive nature, to help me understand my sensitivities for what they really were, or to show me how to channel them in an empowering way, I was left to lean on substances like pornography, alcohol, and promiscuity as my means for coping. I was doing what I could to manage my sensitivity in a highly insensitive world. It was this "self-management," without the guidance of a self-aware, emotionally developed adult, that inevitably led to my fall. I unknowingly robbed myself of my innocence by attempting to manage my sensitivities all on my own. Over time, I even began to despise them for the way they made me feel; hurt, insecure, different, like I didn't belong. No one had ever shown me how to embrace my sensitive nature. No one had ever taught me that my sensitivities were actually a good thing. Yes, you read that correctly. It just so happens that our "sensitivities" are our innate human superpowers.

Each one of us was born gifted. Most of us suppressed our gifts out of fear; fear of being hurt, fear of being different, fear of being cast out, fear of being rejected. All we really wanted when we were young was to feel like we belonged somewhere, so we tried to fit in everywhere. We molded ourselves to our environment thinking it would earn us love and acceptance. Our sensitivities (gifts like intuition, empathy, receptivity, emotional intelligence, and sensory awareness) were always meant to be our unique and special gifts. If they would have been supported, protected, nurtured, and encouraged, especially throughout our young life, we would have naturally learned how to work with them in an empowering way. Almost everything in our young environment told us that our sensitivity was a bad thing. Very early on we learned that our sensitivities made us weak, different from those we loved, especially in a world that seemed to reward the insensitive. Not wanting to feel separate, less than, or unsafe, we suppressed our sensitive nature and conformed. We emulated what we saw in our environment, especially what we saw from our parents.

For me, I was highly empathic as a child. I felt everything. I could effortlessly feel how other people were feeling, even when what they expressed with their words was different from what they were feeling. It was like my body always knew the emotional truth of the situation for all parties involved. When my father would belittle my mother at the dinner table and everyone would laugh, I would feel the undertone of hurt on both sides. I'd feel sick to my stomach. My capacity for emotional empathy was present long before I ever had the words to describe it. My family, like most families, wasn't exactly the textbook definition of "liberated" when it came to emotional or sexual expression. We could talk all day long about what we were doing in life, but never did a conversation start with, "how are you feeling?" This confused me as a child and young man. I often wondered why I felt so much when everyone else seemed to feel so little. It was like I was present to two coexisting yet entirely different worlds, an external world where everyone zoomed around incessantly doing and an internal world where everyone had feelings about what they were doing but never shared them.

The longer this underlying emotional world went unexpressed, the more I questioned its existence. I began to think that maybe there was just something wrong with me, that somehow, I had come out wrong. Maybe God made a mistake when making me. Maybe I was a genetic anomaly and that was why I felt so different from the rest of the world. By the time I hit puberty and my sex energy sprung online, I felt completely overwhelmed by it. Not only was I sensitive and not emotionally equipped to handle the intensity of this primal energy, but I also had no one to talk to about it. For all I knew, I was the only person in the world that felt this way.

I, like all of us, concealed my sensitivity to my creative life force and turned it over into the hands of a $100 billion-dollar entertainment industry to have its way with me. An industry that had zero interest in protecting my innocence. My sensitivity quickly turned into addiction (as it often does), one that ultimately led me down a road of shame. Never was I educated or talked to about sex. No one ever told me about the sacredness and power of my creative life force. I was never given the opportunity to build a constructive, honest, and empowering relationship with my sex energy. I, like all of us, was the product of multiple generations of emotional and sexual repression, the same repression that led to the creation of the porn industry. The only difference being that the porn industry swung all the way from repression to exploitation, and we were all exploited in the process. Our innocence was exploited, and we've been seeking a means to gain it back ever since.

I tell you this story not because I wish for you to blame your parents, our parents' generation, organized religion, or the porn industry for our contemporary era of sexual repression, exploitation, immaturity, superficiality, and violence. It had to go this way in order for us to deeply desire something different. The contrast of our life experience is the fuel for our transformation. Our years of misguided sexual expression and shame were necessary for bringing us to this point in time. All of the sexual confusion, hurt, guilt, and shame that we've felt along the way will now become the raw emotional energy fueling the journey ahead. It goes without saying that we must be one hundred percent responsible for the way it all went; the good, the bad, and the ugly. Don't be fooled, there's much to reconcile. As much as it isn't our fault we ended up this way, it's our responsibility now to reconcile it and make it right.

Healing our superficial relationship to sex is one of the greatest challenges we're up against in the twenty-first century. It's up to us to write a new story. For the first time in our lives, we have all the tools we need to properly breakdown and reconstruct our relationship to sex. Before us lies the opportunity to co-create an entirely new blueprint for every man, woman, and child that will walk in our footsteps. A lot's at stake. If you're reading this now, then you are one of the chosen ones who will plant the early seeds of change and work to nurture them throughout the course of your life. We are here to heal our relationship to sex, starting primarily with ourselves. There's no such thing as an insensitive man. There are only sensitive men and how they learned to channel their sensitivity. Before, we didn't have a choice. Now we do.

Our sons and daughters will not know the trauma of repression because it ends with us. They will grow up with fathers capable of guiding them towards an enlightened relationship with sex, a relationship grounded in unconditional love and rooted in truth. They will know the purity of their hearts, the innocence of their sex energy, and the power within them to channel their creative life force in service to love. We will show them the way by going first. This is the new blueprint. This revolutionary masculine model will liberate our sex energy to serve its highest purpose. It requires your sensitivity. It requires that you call forth that part of you deeply connected to the little ones to come, to the innocence that will be the future inhabitants of Earth. They're following in our footsteps now. How we teach them to relate to their sensitive nature and their sacred sexual life force will determine how life evolves on planet Earth for countless generations to come.

Chapter 2

Over-Sexualized & Sexually Repressed

Let's talk for a moment about our fundamental beliefs about sex and where those beliefs come from. I grew up Catholic, and while my religious upbringing served me in many ways, instilling in me morals like the Golden Rule; do unto others as you would have them do unto you, it failed miserably at preparing me for a lifelong constructive relationship with sex. This is likely the case for many millennials that grew up in religious households. Whether you consider yourself religious, spiritual, agnostic, atheist, reformist, or all around indifferent, religious dogma is at the very heart of our distorted relationship with sex, as well as the shame we've learned to carry around it.

As children, we were raised to believe that we were being watched over and protected by an all knowing God. That felt good to us right up until the point we learned that disobeying Him meant being sent to fiery hell and having our flesh peeled from our bones for all eternity. While our God was a loving God, he was also well aware of our every thought, feeling, and action. He knew not only every time we masturbated, watched porn, fooled around, or had sex, but also every time we thought about masturbating, watching porn, fooling around, or having sex. When it came to sex, God had some pretty strict rules that included:

- Abstinence before marriage
- Celibacy unless procreating
- Prohibition of contraceptive use
- No masturbation, period
- No oral sex, period
- And obviously, no sex (or marriage) between same sex partners

This list might change depending on your faith tradition, but the rule holds. Religion dictated our beliefs around sex. In the Catholic church I grew up in, any funny business outside these rules was strictly forbidden and a sin against the big guy upstairs. If the rules themselves weren't damaging enough, the way they were implemented by our moral authorities certainly did the trick. As all children are, we were naturally curious about our physical body. At some point we stumbled upon the realization that if we touched ourselves a certain way, it felt good. So, naturally, we did. It wasn't until a moral authority, most likely one of our parents, condemned us for innocently sticking our hands down our pants that we learned touching ourselves was bad. "Stop touching yourself like that," or, "get your hands out of your pants." Heaven forbid we were ever discovered touching another child's special parts.

The relationship to sex that we inherited from our moral authorities was based in fear, not love. It's like my pops used to say: his old man put "the fear of God" in him so that when my grandfather was away, my father and his brothers would behave. Religious dogma attempted to do the same thing to us by teaching us to fear being punished by God for our sexual behavior. Not that there aren't religious folks out there that have a very healthy, love-based relationship with sex. I'm certain there are. I'm also certain the people responsible for conveying religious dogma to children most often have good intentions, like protecting children from the practical dangers of sex and not wanting them to make "bad" decisions. Unfortunately, we humans are specially designed for "bad" decisions, especially men. We're different from girls in that we typically have to learn things the hard way. One of our worst decisions to date was choosing to adopt these fear-based rules and make them our own, turning sex into something to fear rather than something to explore consciously.

This created a predicament for us once we hit puberty and

started having sexual thoughts and feelings. We felt conflicted by the ever apparent difference between what we felt in our body and what was being taught to us by the church. Part of us instinctually desired to explore our sexual nature while the other part shamed us for feeling that desire in the first place. That shame, however, was never ours to begin with. Sexual shame is something that was instilled in us by our religious predecessors, not something we were born with. Organized religion, especially those in charge of conveying religious dogma to children, taught us to shame our sexuality, and we've been shaming it all on our own ever since. Even those of us that have long forgotten our religious upbringing can still reflect and remember that shame. The collective discomfort with which we approach the conversation about sex is evidence of its persistence. Sex is the essential process through which new human life is created. In other words, sex is how we all got here. Despite this biological fact, it's rarely ever spoken about openly without the person speaking about it having to feel awkward, uncomfortable, embarrassed, or ashamed. In many ways, it's this collective shame around sex, passed down from one generation to the next, that has kept us up until now from experiencing the full power of our divinely appointed sexual nature.

When I was young, I thought that God looked down on me for my sexual thoughts, feelings, and actions. Every time I masturbated, even without the use of porn, I felt shameful and dirty. I thought God was going to find a way to punish me for being one of his "fallen angels." I expected to be punished. When "bad" things would happen in my life, someone passing away or getting a poor grade on an exam, I would think at least for a moment that this was God's way of punishing me. I remember getting caught in a torrential thunderstorm with my father out in the middle of Black Lake on one of our fishing adventures. The boat's engine had failed. We were left adrift in open water. Lightning flashed down from the heavens as if preceding the four horsemen of the apocalypse, striking the water's surface all around us. Our only option was to weather the storm, taking cover in the small cubbyhole underneath the steering wheel. Shivering from the frigid rain and wind, arms wrapped tightly around my knees, I pinched my eyes closed and started praying. "God, if you get us out of this alive, I promise I'll never masturbate again."

I could have only been about ten at the time. I guess I thought God would save us if I gave him enough leverage to do so, so I pulled out the big guns and made a bargain I was certain he couldn't resist. I had to come up with something, right? After all, our lives were at stake. So, I gave him something I knew would be too good to pass up. Our lives were spared that day, but I didn't keep my end of the bargain. I think I lasted a week. Even though I couldn't help but give in to my sexual appetite, I was growing to despise my sexual predisposition for how it made me feel—unworthy of God's love. Some days I was certain I was doomed to burn in hell for all eternity, right next Satan and all his other loyal subjects. Some days I thought maybe God would spare me out of pity. After all, wasn't it he that made me this way? Most days I tried not to think about it, but that's like asking you not to think about a purple elephant. Good luck with that.

I'd like to think we could do away with all religious dogma as it relates to sex and all of our problems would be solved, but I'm afraid the source of our sexual repression goes back even further than organized religion. Most of our world religions were born out of what we would consider a patriarchal system, not all that unlike the one we live in today. Patriarchy is a social system where men hold the primary power. Men are placed in roles of familial, social, political, and moral authority. Even Jesus, whose teachings have been both idolized and manipulated by many different religions, lived in a patriarchal society. Why do you think religious texts so rarely reference Jesus' beloved,

Mary Magdalene, who was just as much responsible for Jesus' work as he was? When she is mentioned, she's referenced as some kind of hooker or whore. Classic patriarchy. A keynote of any patriarchal system is suppression of the feminine, or in more practical terms, suppression of women. In patriarchal systems, women are considered subordinate to men, usually in "the eyes of God," and most often viewed as the property of men to do with as they please. I could not even begin to recount the evidence for feminine suppression throughout our history as it would require all the remaining text in this book, and then some.

We have a modern-day society that's absolutely obsessed with sex. Sex is everywhere from Internet porn sites to online retail to mass media. Just driving down the road we're liable to see a billboard using sex to advertise, market, or sell us a service or product. And sex, at least in the way it's currently depicted, is something that has been characterized and defined by men in positions of power within patriarchal systems for as long as humans have been recording history. Today, what modern men and women consider sexy, hot, spicy, and erotic, from a cultural perspective, is all something that was originally articulated and defined by men. Men have learned to worship a synthetic feminine of their own creation, one that doesn't even come close to the real thing. Instead, it's all about "Azz N Tittyz," for anyone that listened to Three 6 Mafia as a kid. Oh, and of course, brownie points for having a pretty face. Culturally, we've dumbed down the feminine to a pretty face and a fit body, placing most, if not all of our emphasis on her physical appearance. For those that don't fit this cultural mold, they're left to live on the fringe of society, mostly ignored. For those that do fit the mold, it's a heartless battle to stay at the top, to stay relevant, young, and sexy.

Many women have adapted by molding themselves to meet our culture's patriarchal standards, mostly just trying to make it in a man's world. Hence the dramatic increase in cosmetic plastic surgery over the last two decades, including labiaplasty, thanks to the "picture perfect" vulvas presented in porn. Why are men calling the shots here? That's a great question. Maybe early on we figured out how powerful a fully liberated woman was and decided that wasn't in our best interest. Maybe we thought to ourselves, "we better put a cap on this before it gets out of hand." Or, maybe it was a genetic thing. Maybe men grew to place more cultural value on themselves because their physical structure and strength seemed better suited for a tough and rugged world. Whatever the explanation that got us here, here we are, in a world where patriarchy has externalized our hunger for the real feminine, exploiting women and all that the feminine represents in the process. We've effectively oversexualized everything and sought to satiate our internal hunger for feminine energy through external, mostly distorted means; strip clubs, pornography, prostitution, sex trafficking, sexually explicit material in film, media, music, and more; all under the guise of "harmless entertainment."

Each culture has its own flavor, but if you look closely, you will see that the one consistent element is a fundamentally unrealistic, overly sexualized image of the "ideal woman." Today it looks like a pretty face, round ass, perky breasts (size preference depends on the man), thin waist, all topped by an insatiable sexual appetite like that of a man. If it's not obvious enough already, our modern expression of feminine repression has its roots steeped much deeper than our first introduction to pornography as a teenager. Feminine suppression, sexual repression, and sexual exploitation are quite literally woven into the fabric of our human history, through religious dogma and the patriarchal systems it was born out of. This may not be headlined in history books or openly explored in modern news, but these core themes have operated in the background of human culture for as long as we've been documenting history.

When I say the journey of restoring the heart into human sexuality is bigger than any one of us alone, I mean it. I'm not meaning to belittle our personal histories. I'm inviting us into understanding them within the greater context of our collective history.

We're all part of a system that we'd better become aware of, because our participation in it keeps it going. My belief is that we've all been both men and women in other lifetimes. We've all been the abusers and the abused. This isn't a story of men versus women, the battle of the sexes, or who's right and who's wrong in terms of the appropriate expression of our sexuality. It's a story of reconciliation. It's a story of once again balancing the divine poles of masculine and feminine energy within ourselves, each other, and the world. As we liberate this feminine energy in both men and women, restoring it to its rightful place in society, we also restore our collective human heart, not only in relationship to sex, but in relationship to every other area of life as well. Honoring the feminine is one hundred percent necessary for truly embodying the qualities of the divine masculine. In fact, embracing our inner-feminine is actually *how* we become fully embodied in our sacred masculine. Balancing these energies is what will allow us to reestablish right relations between men and women.

Prior to starting my heart-opening journey, I had participated in personal and professional development courses for nearly three years. My mind was well developed in viewing my emotions as meaningless, other than the meaning I gave to them. For years I was trained to view my emotions as nothing more than physiological fluctuations in body chemistry that I applied meaning to. I one hundred percent know what it's like to be disconnected from my inner-feminine, to be disconnected from my emotional body. I too had to make the long journey from my head to my heart.

Men are warriors at heart, but until we embrace our ability to feel and feel deeply, we'll have no idea what it is we're fighting for. As men, we were never shown how to properly feel and express our emotions. Most of us have gone our entire lives bottling up our hurt because we're terrified of feeling it. The idea of death is more enticing to us than the thought of being emotionally vulnerable. Learning to express my heart with my emotions wasn't something that came naturally to me. When I started my heart-opening journey, I could barely describe to you with words what I was feeling emotionally, let alone allow my body to express it freely. I was so deeply entrenched in my mind that my body was only capable of expressing emotions like frustration, anger, resentment, and rage. Over time it became easier to allow my body to express other emotions, but it was especially challenging in the beginning.

Over the last two and a half years, I gave myself full permission to dive into my emotional body, exploring its depth, dynamism, and darkness. Don't worry, I'm still a man, and you will be too when it's all said and done. No one's trying to turn you into a woman here. What I've learned from my journey is that genuine, open-hearted, authentic, and vulnerable emotional expression is one of the most important things the men of our time can learn. There is nothing more liberating than being able to express an emotion as is rises, rather than having to exert so much energy towards keeping it down. It's way better than getting stuck with an unexpressed emotion inside for days, weeks, months, even years. Heaven only knows how many moments of delight, freedom, connection, and intimacy we've missed because of trapped emotions. This journey has allowed me to release three decades worth of unexpressed emotions. Underneath them was all the passion, energy, creativity, and health I had been looking for. I wish I could get back all that money I spent on energy supplements.

I know the idea of exploring what we've emotionally repressed might seem threatening, but I assure you, you have nothing to lose and everything to gain. If we're willing to embrace the inner qualities we currently shun, our inner-feminine, we at least give ourselves the opportunity to see how senseless it is for us to try and fill our hunger for the feminine through women and sex. Not only that, but we give our physical bodies permission to let go of all the emotional baggage we've been carrying our entire lives. It's only scary at first because it's unknown. It feels foreign, given our upbringing and cultural conditioning told us that any man connected to his emotional body is gay. Once again, our religious upbringing did a great job of having us fear that. If you lean in just enough, you'll discover what it is you are looking for.

I feel more liberated at thirty years old than I have at any other point in my life because I intentionally leaned into this process of opening up my heart and embracing those inner-feminine qualities I had done everything I could to stamp out. Through it, I've discovered what true masculinity is to me; protecting the innocence, honoring the feminine, and defending the sacred. Along the way I got to rediscover my creative side, a side of me I thought never existed to begin with. I also discovered how to unconditionally love, accept, honor, and hold massive space for the feminine in both men and women. I've witnessed first-hand how healing it can be for a woman to be around a man that's embodied in his feminine, and therefore his masculine. Something in the energetics of the exchange immediately goes to work on healing our long history of feminine suppression.

It's tremendously rewarding work, but it doesn't come without sacrifice, the first being our willingness to let go of our ego's understanding of masculinity. I get that this probably won't resonate with everyone, but for those with whom it does, believe me when I say that you are finally safe to be who you really are, sensitivities and all, and be fully loved for it. You are still that masculine warrior. In fact, you had to be to get here. The more we honor and embrace the feminine within ourselves, the more we balance the polarities between the masculine and the feminine in our world. This will ultimately look like a more compassionate, peaceful, and harmonious existence for all beings on our planet.

I will say it again: men are warriors at heart, but until we embrace our ability to feel and feel deeply, embodying our own inner feminine, we'll have no idea what we're fighting for. This breeds anger and aggression without purpose. When we allow the slow death of the feminine within us, we subsequentially sequester our inner fire, our passion, our depth, and our connection to our purpose. Without these things we are nothing. It is true that masculinity bestows masculinity, but the purest expression of masculine energy can only ever flow through an open and receptive heart. Reopening our heart requires us to feel what's kept it closed. This is just one of the many ways in which the feminine serves the masculine; "she" reminds us of what it is we're fighting for… love.

Chapter 3

Sex Energy

Our sex energy is one of our greatest gifts and hands down one of the most powerful creative forces in all of the Universe. It was intentionally gifted to us by our creator as our means for fully exploring our human capacity for creativity. We were given permission to create as we wished, fully trusted to wield this power wisely. On the most fundamental level, our sex energy generates the necessary internal forces for one person to unite with another and procreate new human life; an inherently miraculous process. Many things had to unfold perfectly over the course of millennia for you to be born, for you to be here now, reading this material.

Sex energy is the fundamental energy with which we were all created. It's the fundamental energy with which each of us will go on creating until evolution directs us otherwise. Sex energy is the energy of creation itself, synonymous with what some might call our creative life force, prana, chi, or kundalini. Our sex energy does so much more than simply help us reach climax. When liberated and intentionally circulated through an open heart, our sex energy has the power to heal emotional wounds, ignite our entire body with pleasure, revitalize our spiritual/energetic body, expand our creative potential, and merge our personal awareness with that of cosmic consciousness. It's how we create entirely new realities or perpetuate the ones already in existence.

On a not so fundamental level, at least in the sense that most of us were never taught this, our sex energy is capable of conceiving more than just a physical child. It can help us conceive ideas, visions, insights and inspired actions that eventually lead to creative endeavors like passion projects, social movements, mission driven businesses, and more. Sex energy is a magical force, a mystical energy that frightens many because of its potency. Rightfully so given the harm that can come when it's used manipulatively, or by someone that has yet to connect this energy with their heart. It takes a truly embodied man to stand in his sexual power, heart wide open, and consciously wield his sex energy for good.

As men, we interact with this energy every single day, yet its use is mostly dictated by our unconscious conditioning. Being one of the most creative forces in the entire Universe, our sex energy is doing what it does best virtually 24/7, 365 days a year, creating! But *what* it's being used to create is what actually matters. Make no mistake, our awareness of this energy and how we choose to channel it absolutely matters. When circulated with an open heart, our sex energy goes to work creating more love in the world. When circulated in response to fear, power dynamics, manipulation, or our conditioned sexual impulses like the ones we received from porn, our sex energy goes to work creating more fear, objectification, dehumanization, cruelty, and separation in the world, further veiling our interconnectedness.

Let's clarify some things. We're obviously talking about two different but related things here; sex and sex energy. Sex is obviously that thing we do with our physical bodies. It's as simple as all of the right parts going in all of the right places. Our sex energy on the other hand is the energy we *feel* in our body as the magic is happening; those heightened sensations, that ecstatic stirring, those tingly vibrations that manifest as goosebumps on our skin. That, my friends, is our sex energy. This may come as a surprise to you, but we don't actually need to be having sex in order to access this abundance of creative energy. This is where most men get tripped up. We can feel those same orgasmic sensations that we experience during sex while doing other "non-sexual" things like singing, dancing, performing, doing breathwork, or working on a creative project.

Probably the best non-sexual example of this is listening to music, those moments when the beat drops and hits you on a somatic level. It's that, "OMG I'm so lit right now I feel like I could fly" kind of feeling. That's your sex energy. As much as it might seem like we need something outside of us to stimulate this energy, like turning on a porn video and instantly feeling aroused, it's actually the other way around. Our sex energy is always, already present within our physical body and we are the ones that inspire its arousal through our intentions, attention, and awareness. Whether we realize it or not, we have absolute control over how, when, and in response to what this energy becomes active. We are the ones that stimulate and circulate this energy from within, rather than being the victims of anything outside of us. That's an incredibly important awareness to have in terms of reclaiming our power. However, most men were never taught about their sex energy, let alone made familiar with it enough to practice circulating it consciously. Instead of empowering us, it scares us because it's intense and seemingly uncontrollable.

Interesting thing, arousal, isn't it? When something captures and arouses our sex energy, we feel alive inside. It's like our bodies jump from a 110V power outlet source to a 240V in a matter of seconds. Suddenly we are catapulted into what feels like an endless abyss of raw, primal energy that typically lasts for as long as we entertain it. For men, what currently activates our sex energy is mostly sex; sexual imagery, sexual thoughts, daydreams about sex, seeing an attractive woman and fantasizing about having sex with her, and essentially over sexualizing just about any normal, everyday life experience. Yes, there is the occasional "morning wood," as well as those erections caused by nothing more than simple friction, but I'm not talking about that here.

I'm talking about the circulation of our sex energy being an unconscious byproduct of our conditioning. We have unintentionally conditioned ourselves to circulate our sex energy in response to synthetic, artificial, and imitation stimuli. Much of the commercial world already knows this, especially those interested in selling you on your imperfections. This is why you see overly sexualized imagery virtually everywhere being used as a means to advertise, market, and sell you things. If they can arouse your sex energy while you peek through a magazine, watch television, or drive past a billboard, then you'll be unconsciously inclined to pay more attention to what they're selling. Culturally, at least in the West and in other parts of the developed world, this sales tactic has been entirely normalized.

Sex is only one very small part of our lives. Yet somehow, at least for men, it seems to occupy most of our attention, certainly more than it merits given what a small percentage of our time we actually spend having sex. My point is, what if we could learn how to consciously control when, where, with whom, and towards what our sex energy was activated, circulated, and directed? What if we could learn how to consciously direct it towards creating those things that we really, truly desire? Imagine feeling aroused in the same way you are by a sexual fantasy by a creative vision that inspires you. Maybe it's that business you've always dreamt of starting or seeing yourself on stage speaking in front of thousands. Maybe you dream of a planet with clean oceans and thriving natural ecosystems. Imagine feeling that same rush of energy, that same 110V to 240V feeling and channeling it towards the innovative solutions that will inevitably protect and sustain all oceanic and terrestrial life on Earth. Imagine for a moment that the arousal you felt in response to this creative inspiration was just as pleasurable to you as sex. Imagine it being more pleasurable and lasting for hours, maybe even days, much longer than a brief boulevard to ejaculation.

It's good to remember here that most of us were never really given a chance to cultivate an empowering relationship with our sex energy. We learned very early on that sex was bad unless it was happening between married couples as a means to make a baby. Our genetics obviously shared a different perspective. No one ever taught us about our sex energy; what it was, what it could be used for, why our bodies suddenly felt so different, how to channel it constructively, or how to properly manage our primal sex drive that seemed to spring up overnight. If our sex energy and overall sexual nature really was a gift from God, then why were our religious leaders, parents, school systems, and authority figures teaching us otherwise? Why were we raised to fear our sex energy rather than embrace it for its inherently powerful, creative nature?

If you can teach a young man to repress and shame his most potent means of creative expression, as opposed to provide him with an education and a structure to properly channel it, then you can effectively control him. The complexity of mental and emotional confusion that follows sexual repression severs men from their true source of inner power, leaving them at the mercy of whomever might wish to control them. Organized religion is a great example of this. Teach men to deny their innate sexual nature, instill shame as their internal referee, provide an external structure like the Holy Bible as a means for their salvation, and voila, you've got yourself power and influence. Repress sex, instill shame, offer a solution, gain power and influence.

Puberty is an extremely sensitive time for most boys, the time when our bodies develop into their physical maturity, a time when our hormone levels shift and change. Suddenly we feel different about pretty much everything in our lives; ourselves, our family, our friends, and especially women. Seemingly overnight, we become irritable towards our parents and siblings and disinterested in all the things that we used to love as a kid. It's almost as if this energy begins changing nearly every aspect of our lives, long before we're ever equipped mentally or emotionally to handle it. For those of you who are not men, the feeling within a man's body of this primal awakening, the awakening of his sex energy, is not something that's experienced subtly. For those of us that did not have good role models or a proper support system in place, this energy quickly overwhelmed us. Given all that we had heard from our parents, authority figures, educators, and religious leaders about sex, we were already coming from a place of fear to begin with.

Add in the fact that emotional expression was not taught or valued in our family household and it only made sense that we resorted to porn to educate ourselves and find a "release" for this energy. The obvious problem is that the porn industry exploited this sensitive situation. By design, it was created to lure us with its flashing lights, shiny objects, and promises of splendor, safety, and education, only to spit us out years later, far from our innocent beginnings. We were being used, all of us, by forces and systems of which we are still a part.

Our inner innocence was not so innocently lured into this well-oiled, well-established, sex energy siphoning system. Each time we plugged in, turned on our computer screen and took in this imagery, our physical biochemistry responded to the artificial stimuli as if it were the real thing, real life sex with another human being. In those moments, not only was our sex energy activated as we entered into that well-researched "porn trance," but it was also devoted to co-creating something entirely bankrupt. The simultaneous drop of dopamine into our neurophysiology, along with a whole host of other reward chemicals, sealed the deal. The addictive pleasure cycle kept us coming back for more. As our porn usage continued, the relationship between our sex energy and this synthetic reality strengthened, as did the neurological pathways being carved into our brain.

We should have been taught that our sex energy is sacred and one of the most powerful creative forces in all of the Universe, something to be used intentionally and channeled towards those creative expressions that mean the most to us. Instead, we simply learned to stimulate our superficial sex organs and settle for a momentary glimpse into the true potential of this energy. Instead of learning how our sex energy could go to work towards bringing to life all of our biggest and most heartfelt dreams, we simply offered it up to be manipulated, twisted, and poisoned. It stays this way for most men throughout their entire lives because the sad reality is, most of us never overcome this biochemical addiction. Most of us continue to drink the poison without realizing we're sick. Most men are never offered the opportunity to reclaim their sexual innocence. We never actually learn about the broken system we're a part of, let alone our innate ability to constructively channel our own creative life force in a way that serves love rather than dehumanization.

We all know the rest of the story all too well because we've lived it. Here we are, adult men, feeling in our hearts a genuine desire to go deeper into our sexual nature, deeper into real intimacy, deeper into our relationship with this powerful creative energy, yet we're deeply trapped by our lifelong patterns, practices, and biochemical addictions. We've been drinking the poison for so long that it's seeped into our bones. What the hell do we do now? How in God's name are we going to undo what's been done, break free from the addictive cycle, heal our superficial relationship to sex, and create an entirely new relationship with our sexuality that's based on love instead of fear? Just as someone with heavy metal poisoning has to cleanse and detox their body to rid themselves of what's ailing them, we too have to cleanse and detox our mind and body. We need to muster up all of the energy we have to fight for our innocence, but we first ought to get real with ourselves about whether or not we're up for the battle.

If Lao Tzu is correct and the journey of a thousand miles does in fact begin with a single step, the first step of this journey will require ruthless honesty, integrity, strength of heart, and a willingness to take this journey on as our primary method for healing our collective sex trauma. Step one is becoming acutely aware of all the areas in our lives where our sex energy is currently hooked by our conditioning, leaking, and not serving to love. I have spoken a lot about porn, but porn is not the addiction for every man. For some it's womanizing, objectification, seduction, promiscuity, one night stands, or sexual manipulation for their own selfish gain. This can be the most challenging step, as our entire lives have been constructed around a false understanding of who we are sexually. Yes, this means unplugging the porn, abstaining from sex where we use women and discard them, hookups under the influence of alcohol or other substances, masturbation to unconscious, sexual imagery, ejaculation for the sole purpose of "getting off," and putting our sex energy onto women that don't desire it. Maybe for you it's taking it a step further and turning off the television for a while, going off social media, cutting out the drinking, and disconnecting from those people, places, and things that cause you to feel bad for reasons you can't yet name.

If you really do intend to return to your true, innocent, and original sexual nature, then you're going to have to commit to some serious work in removing from your environment all of those things that continuously manipulate your mind, hijack your physiology, and keep you small, both for yourself and for the world. Otherwise, this whole process will be like learning how to sail in a boat with dozens of cracks in its baseboards. Rather than learning to sail, we'll waste all of our time and energy bailing out the boat. Before heading out into open water, it's important we spend the necessary time on land, addressing our vessel's integrity. That way, by the time we're out on the open water, we'll be free to learn and enjoy the experience of sailing. Not to say that things won't come up. Inevitably, they will, as we all know nature can be unpredictable at times. But when they do, we'll be prepared, trained, and ready to address them head on.

Our sex energy is worthy and deserving of our upmost attention, reverence, and respect. It was gifted to us as our birthright, to receive the innocence of pleasure while simultaneously co-creating a world deeply rooted in love. The way our sex energy is already hooked and the real-life impact of that is currently creating anything but love. When we masturbate to porn or engage in heartless sex, getting our fix and really nothing more, we are left with an internal hunger that cannot be satisfied through external means. What we have is never enough and what we do to satisfy ourselves externally comes at a tremendous cost. We consume unconsciously, attempting to satiate the hunger, our actions at the expense of others. As men, we use porn, masturbation, and sex to mask our loneliness, prove our masculinity (primarily to ourselves), distract us from our suffering, to feel some sense of connection to the feminine we're suppressing internally, and to avoid having to see, feel, and receive who we really are, how loved we truly are, and the bigness of our mission and purpose.

If we created the old way of doing things, we can create a new way that serves everyone involved. We can use our sex energy to co-create intimacy, unconditional love, devotion, transparency, truth, passion, and the feelings of being deeply seen and known; all things that actually do fulfill us on the inside and allow us to show up powerfully for ourselves and others. Step one is unplugging from all the distractions that keep us unconsciously hooked into our outdated conditioning.

I'm convinced that the reality of you channeling your sex energy in this way is far more satisfying than you can imagine. It for sure has been for me. The integrity I have with myself and my own creative life force propels me to show up in life as a fiercely passionate, loving man. It's no joke, like being a modern-day superhero disguised as an average Joe. There came a point in time where I had to choose for real what kind of man I was going to be, the kind of man that led personal and professional development programs while still watching porn, objectifying women, cheating on his girlfriends, sleeping around, and using his sex energy for his own personal gain, no matter what the consequences, or the type of man that chose to come clean with his lack of integrity and clean it up; for his future wife's sake, for his future children's sake, for humanity's sake, and most importantly, for the sake of his own heart.

Trust me, it's not about being perfect. It most definitely is about being honest and real, starting with ourselves. Once you tap into the true potency and power of your sex energy, there will be no going back for you. Your entire life will be given by the integrity with which you wield it. Rarely are we ever fully aware of the actual depth of our own programming until we pause long enough to take a good look. More than likely, if you're still masturbating to porn or chasing one-night stands, your conditioning is operating your sex energy anytime your mind isn't being forced to focus on something else.

I'll leave you here with a bit of inspiration to contemplate as we intentionally set sail into the coming chapters. Some of the most beautiful experiences I've had in receiving the purity and potency of my sex energy has been through music. These artists are examples of human beings that have mastered their ability to channel their sex energy in a way that opens the hearts of others. Snatam Kaur Khalsa is a perfect example of such a person. When I listen to her songs, my sex energy dances the dance of the divine. Love overcomes me as my heart relaxes into remembering its purest essence. Listen to her song, Ong Namo, before moving on. You can find it easily on YouTube. It will be a shining example for you to remember your purity as we reawaken to our sexual innocence.

It can be easy to get wrapped up in the thwarted expressions of human sexuality, but it's often far more rewarding to focus on how much it is already being used for good. It all comes back down to the heart. If our heart is open, we will inevitably channel our sex energy with love. As we move on to the next section and begin diving into eliminating the things that distract our creative life force, don't forget that at our core, we were designed to channel our sex energy in service to love. In fact, at its core, sex energy *is* love, the love of the divine flowing through our physical form. We are blessed to have been given such a loving power. Expanding our awareness around its misguided use will only empower us to draw back to ourselves more of our displaced sex energy, returning it once again to love. This isn't a game of shame or self-pity. This is the inspired mission of delivering the most powerful creative energy in the Universe back into the hands of love.

Chapter 4

Clearing Your Slate

It's obvious by now that I come down pretty hard on the porn industry, and rightfully so. When you know something is siphoning your creative life force, robbing you of real intimacy, stunting your true sexual power, dropping your vibration, and contributing to the global demand for sex trafficking and human slavery… I think you get what I'm saying here. How we respond becomes a matter of behavioral integrity and standing for what we know to be right and good in our heart. When we know better, we do better, and that includes taking a good clean look at all of the areas in our life where our sex energy is currently leaking out to people and things that are not in service to love.

Pornography is one of those things. But, as you will soon find out, quitting porn won't be enough for you to create the kind of relationship with your sex energy that I'm talking about here. It's certainly a start, but the way in which this industry has programmed our neural networks extends far beyond masturbating in front of a computer screen. Our entire lives have been constructed around a false understanding of our sexuality, the impact of which has been devastating. This isn't something we can put a cultural band aid on and change overnight. It's a fundamental human issue, one that must be addressed inside each one of us. Even if you were to quit watching porn today, in this very moment, it would still continue to impact your psyche for years. I know this because I've been porn free now for over three years and there are still times when the porn programming tries to capture my awareness. Old habits die hard, but they must die in order for new ones to be born in their place.

The dawn of social media exploded our capacity for social connection. In today's world, we can quite literally be anywhere on Earth and maintain some sense of digital connection with the people in our lives. It's truly incredible. It's also incredible how social media can be utilized to create true social impact. It's a fantastic platform for sharing our passions and creative expressions with the world. As media has evolved, so has the frequency of our social media platforms. Recalling how our minds have been trained through decades of pornography use to sexually objectify women, and how centuries of feminine suppression has led to women in many ways sexually objectifying themselves, continually altering their physical appearance to meet the standards of what our patriarchal culture deems "sexy," we can easily see how all of this plays out in our artificial reality called social media.

Social media has become the new porn. While we may not see explicitly pornographic images on social media platforms like Instagram or Facebook, what we do see really isn't that much different from porn. For instance, right now, if I really wanted to, I could hop on Instagram and within seconds be viewing a virtually unlimited supply of naked women with their nipples and vulvas scribbled out. If that wasn't appealing enough, I could always peruse through the everlasting list of aspiring Victoria's Secret models; clothed, of course, but just barely enough to inspire the imagination. Okay, let's say I was feeling really lazy. In this case, I could simply login and wait long enough for the inevitable "bot" to solicit my inbox with an invitation to view her naked photos over on her "private website."

Hear me out here, I am in no way saying that people should not be free to express their sensuality/sexuality however they see fit, in whatever way feels right to them. I fiercely believe that each one of us reserves the sovereign right to express ourselves in whatever way we are genuinely guided. My point in sharing this is to let you know that the same thing that happens when a man flips open his laptop and starts watching porn is now happening every time he logs into his social media account and starts looking at photos of women. His sex energy gets activated and unconsciously projected out onto those women he sees while scrolling. This habit perpetuates the same conditioning that he received from watching porn, while further distracting him from channeling his sex energy in a truly empowering way. While it's not anyone else's responsibility to manage how a man chooses to channel his sex energy, other than that man himself, it is something I feel would be wise for us all to become aware of.

Our sexuality is most safely expressed inside a container that's equipped to honor such expressions as sacred. For me, Instagram and other social media platforms like it, simply aren't containers that are capable of protecting us in that way. It's no secret really, everyday men all over the world pull out their penis and masturbate to photos they see on social media. I apologize for being brash, but it's something that must be addressed if we're going to continue utilizing these platforms. Everyday men and women use this sexual hyperactivity to their own advantage; to gain followers, sell products, receive validation, and expand their "influence." It's obviously working, the only question being, what is it working towards? More of the same? Or towards establishing a new, more empowered, and sacred relationship with sex?

It doesn't stop with social media either. Every time a man steps out into the world that same pornographic mentality goes with him. We find ourselves unconsciously objectifying women, checking them out, looking them up and down, judging them as attractive or not attractive, and determining rather immediately whether or not we would have sex with them. It happens at the grocery store, at the gas pump, the gym, restaurants, bars, clubs; hell, it even happens just driving down the street. All day long this programming runs just outside of our conscious awareness.

Whether we're aware of it or not, this programming is very much impacting our in-the-moment ability to focus our energy on the things that actually matter to us. 99.9999999% of the time, nothing ever comes of these subconscious fantasies, as in we never actually have a sexual encounter with those women. Over and over again we simply fuel the same superficial stimulation that more than likely will have us go and release on our own. As much as our mind likes to play at fantasy, our reality tells a much different story. Frankly, as a thirty-year-old man committed to making a real and lasting impact in the world, I'm far more interested in what we can create with our sex energy as opposed to pursuing every sexual fantasy to its very meaningless end. You feel me? I say this with compassion and a profound understanding of our inherited and cognitive conditioning, but all of this is just one giant distraction keeping us from actually pursuing what we came here to do.

This is a very intentional and clear invitation to you to take considerable action today towards eliminating the real-life distractions that cause you to unconsciously and consistently leak your sex energy. Why? So that we can collectively reconnect with our sex energy in a way that serves us rather than harms us. Start by eliminating porn and then expand your efforts from there. Take a ruthless look at your social media platforms and unfollow the people, organizations, and entities that have you emptying yourself of your creative life force. If you're the one triggering this porn response, dial back your efforts. Notice where you're using your sex energy to take advantage of others. Maybe even take a break from social media all together, providing you the opportunity to take that energy that's constantly being projected outward and focus it inward on yourself. The real world, your internal world, has so much more to offer you in terms of genuine fulfillment and satisfaction.

Continuing onward, cut out the alcohol, at least in the quantities that have you stoop into old, unconscious, and programmed behaviors. You and I both know alcohol changes us, even if, appearance wise, it seems to make us this carefree, stress-less, happy-go-lucky guy. Caffeine, Westerners' drug of choice, stimulates the sympathetic nervous system putting us into a fight, flight, or freeze response. It triggers mental overactivity, meaning it amplifies preexisting mental patterning. Cut it out or reduce it dramatically. I had no idea how over-taxed and over-stimulated by body was until I removed caffeine from my diet, a chemical I consumed every day, multiple times a day, for over ten years of my life. Nicotine also aggravates the nervous system to release adrenaline, your body's physiological response to fear. Chuck it. We're looking to slow down and calm the nervous system, not speed it up, so we can better access our unconscious patterning. All of these chemicals give our conditioning a foothold on us.

With these actions alone you've already taken back a substantial amount of energy that's typically getting wasted every day. Go ahead and turn off the television while you're at it, mass media being a primary reinforcing agent for our false understanding of our sexuality. Remember, sex sells, and at this stage in our human evolution, it's all about the almighty dollar. Mainstream media will undoubtedly do its best to arouse you, yet keep you just unsatisfied enough to keep coming back for more. Think about it, you turn on the "tell-a-vision," flip to a "channel," and receive "programming." The same goes for YouTube, Netflix, Zulu, Amazon Video. Only you know where your sex energy is leaking. Clean it up. Be ruthlessly honest with yourself. Get an accountability partner.

As you clear these low frequency habits, you'll start to expand your awareness around when and where your sex energy gets activated, what that feels like in your body, and how your mind typically responds with its fantasies. Just notice this. It's not something to engage with in any way, unless of course you're out to make your life a living hell. Your awareness of how your patterns play out is more than enough to start creating the necessary foundation for change. Don't fight them and don't go to battle with them in your mind. If you attempt to suppress, label, judge, or condemn them, you'll only generate more shame. The tendency can be to take a train that's going 200 miles an hour in one direction (our current sexual conditioning) and try to make it do a complete 180 in less than three seconds. De-conditioning takes time. Most of us have been unconsciously practicing these superficial patters for at least a decade, so it's only logical that it's going to take some time to rewire our brain chemistry.

They say that neurons that fire together wire together, well these ones have been firing together since puberty. It's primarily through our awareness of our conditioning and our unbiased observation of it that we begin the de-conditioning process. When your mind gets activated in response to your sex energy being stimulated, just witness it. Rather than indulging in it unconsciously or responding to it with shame, disengage and witness it from one step behind your mental awareness. This is called being the Observer. Let your awareness expand just far enough to allow you to witness your mind's sexual immaturity without having to do anything about it. It's simply programming that you adopted playing itself out in the way that it always has with the entire force of our collective genetic and cultural past fueling it. You were not the you that you are now when you first adopted it. You are, however, the you that you are now. For that reason, you are absolutely capable of using your awareness to witness your mind "in the act."

Our awareness of our sex energy, as it becomes activated within us, allows us to create a degree of internal separation between us (who we really are) and whatever way our mind and body have adapted to react to external stimuli. When we take a step back and observe it happening, we can actually experience with full awareness how our physiology has been hijacked by these patterns of objectification, fantasy, repression, and shame. When we start to see the bigger picture, we can actually understand that our innocence was stolen from us before we were ever capable of protecting it. We can see how one of our strongest primal instincts was manipulated by "the powers that be" and used against us as a means to keep us suppressed, confused, distracted, and small. When that awareness sinks in, removing these distractions becomes an act of rebellion, a revolutionary act of stepping out of this broken system and stepping into our sovereignty. As our awareness expands further, we'll be able to see just how far and wide this manipulation has spread into the mass consciousness of humanity, and therefore, our essential role in reconciling it. Anything we do for ourselves, any old conditionings we resolve, patterns we release, wounds we heal, we do for all of humanity. What I heal and transform within me I also heal and transform within the world.

The number one objection I hear from men when it comes to quitting porn is something along the lines of, "it's harmless," as in, "how I choose to channel my sex energy and express my sexuality doesn't impact anyone other than me." To which I politely reply, "bullshit." Just as every dollar we spend is our vote for the continual supply of a specific product or service, every time we sexually objectify a woman in any way, shape, or form, we place our vote for more dehumanization. We say, "yes, thank you. I'll have some more of that, please!" While that may seem harmless to you now as the one placing the vote, imagine another man just like you voting for the dehumanization of someone you love, say your daughter. Imagine your daughter innocently stepping out into the world and receiving all of those votes, becoming a metaphorical polling station for the "harmless" affairs of men. Imagine this happening in her schools, workplaces, online environments, social media platforms, recreational spaces, gyms, grocery stores, retail centers and so on from the day she hits puberty onward for the rest of her life.

Now look me in my eyes and tell me that how we choose to channel our sex energy is harmless.

It's often easy for us to think of the old, sleazy, wrinkly men that smoke cigars and drink bourbon on the rocks as the "perpetrators." It's often much more challenging for us to see ourselves, the clean cut, well dressed, well educated, successful, attractive young men as the perpetrators. I would know, I was one of them. We do this virtually all day, every day, fooling ourselves into believing that it's all somehow harmless. When in reality, it's this normalized aspect of our patriarchal society that allows men to consistently, energetically violate women. Not to say that it doesn't go the other way around, women objectifying men, but I think you recognize what I'm conveying here.

I asked my friend, Ashley, an anti-trafficking advocate in Phoenix, AZ, to speak to the "harmless" connection between pornography, strip clubs, prostitution, and sex trafficking. Here is what she shared:

As you can imagine, it is really difficult to get an honest pulse on the reality of how many individuals are being sexually exploited or trafficked in pornography and in the stripping industry. There are a couple of nonprofits that do a good job of trying to pin down these statistics. Understandably, many victims of trafficking/exploitation either don't report out of fear or are so brainwashed they don't realize they are being trafficked/exploited. Meaning the statistics they do have are likely much lower than reality.

We worked with a girl here in Phoenix who was a stripper and in confidence she told us that at the strip club she worked at, every girl had a pimp, meaning none of the money a girl made was taken home for herself. At other clubs, they have a pretty strict policy that the girls cannot do anything more than dance. Usually at clubs where girls have pimps, they will offer full service (off the radar of course). Many of the girls are likely underage due to the demand for full nudity, most patrons preferring very young girls.

There is a pretty informative documentary about the porn industry on Netflix called Hot Girls Wanted. It shows a glimpse into how desperate many of the girls are when they get into the industry and how they are often taken advantage of. Then you have the fact that the industry is highly unregulated, so people who make porn can be severely taken advantage of and lied to about what they are making.

There was a recent settlement in CA for $12 million that a woman won against a porn company for lying to her about how her content was going to be sold. And then you get into the fact that the deeper and more perverted porn gets, it fuels a demand for child porn.

To further expand on Ashley's statement, I dug up some shocking consumer statistics prepared by the National Center on Sexual Exploitation and hosted on Fight the New Drug's website. Here are just a few:

- 64% of young people, ages 13–24, actively seek out pornography weekly or more often.
- A study of 14- to 19-year-olds found that females who consumed pornographic videos were at a significantly greater likelihood of being victims of sexual harassment or sexual assault.
- A Swedish study of 18-year-old males found that frequent consumers of pornography were significantly more likely to have sold and bought sex than other boys of the same age.
- A 2015 meta-analysis of 22 studies from seven countries found that internationally the consumption of pornography was significantly associated with increases in verbal and physical aggression, among males and females alike.
- A recent UK survey found that 44% of males aged 11–16 who consumed pornography reported that online pornography gave them ideas about the type of sex they wanted to try.
- Porn sites receive more regular traffic each month than

Netflix, Amazon, and Twitter combined.
- 35% of all Internet downloads are porn-related.
- 34% of Internet users have been exposed to unwanted porn via ads, pop-ups, etc.
- The "teen" porn category has topped porn site searches for the last six years.
- At least 30% of all data transferred across the Internet is porn-related.
- The most common female role stated in porn titles is that of women in their 20s portraying teenagers.
- Recorded child sexual exploitation (known as "child porn") is one of the fastest-growing online businesses.
- 624,000+ child porn traders have been discovered online in the U.S.
- Between 2005 and 2009, child porn was hosted on servers located in all 50 states.
- Porn is a global, estimated $97 billion industry, with about $12 billion of that coming from the U.S.
- The world's largest free porn site received over 33,500,000,000 visits during 2018 alone.

So, think about your daughter(s), present or future, your sisters, your partners, your mothers, and how you would feel if they became the victims of sexual exploitation. Remember them as you do your part in eliminating all the areas of your life in which your sex energy is leaking. Realistically, every woman we objectify is a daughter to someone, possibly a sister, a partner, or a mother herself, her innocence the victim of our unconscious behaviors.

Ideally, looking through this lens will have you take this process a little bit more seriously. We have the power to change the course of history through our awareness of our sex energy and our aligned action of addressing its leaks. Dig deep and decide right now what kind of man you're committed to being, for yourself, your beloved, your children, your communities, and the world. Then, align the use of your sex energy with that decision rather than what's already been decided for you up until now. It's not about being perfect. It's about being human as fuck, while at the same time, doing everything in our power to protect and honor what's sacred in all of us.

Chapter 5

Raising Your Vibration

Vibration is a tricky subject. No one really knows what you mean when you say it, but everyone already has their own preconceived notion of what it means to them. What I mean when I say we're going to raise our vibration is simple. I mean we're going to improve the quality of energy emanating from our body. We're going to shift our energy from where it is now to an energy closer to that of our higher-self. Don't worry, I'll explain "higher-self" later on in this chapter. We can call this energy our vibration, our frequency, our come from, our aura, or simply the energetic impact we have on ourselves and those around us. I'm going to call it our vibration, because that's the way I like to think about it.

There are many different energy sources to choose from when it comes to powering your home. You could choose coal, petroleum, natural gas, solar, or wind to name a few. The quality of energy produced from burning coal is much different to the quality of energy produced from capturing the sun's radiation. One requires clearing robust acreages of land, heavy machinery to dig into the Earth's surface, destruction of natural habitat, environmental pollution of air, water, and land, and results in carbon dioxide being released into the atmosphere, contributing to the devastating effects of climate change. The other requires a few simple raw materials, manufacturing, installation, and voila, an endless supply of clean energy that's good for us and good for the environment. When you flip the light switch on in your kitchen, both result in the kitchen lights coming on, but both have a very different impact on you and the world around you. Our vibration is similar. It's the subtle, behind the scenes energy that we emanate that can cause a desirable or an undesirable impact on us and the world around us.

Through our awareness, we have the ability to influence how high or low we "vibe" in any given moment. We can choose the quality of our energy, whether we're more like coal or more like solar. Activities like writing a list of gratitudes, eating healthily, drinking ceremonial-grade cacao, meditating, dancing, breath-work, love-making, grounding barefoot on the Earth's surface, going out into nature, exercising, swimming in the ocean, doing creative right-brain activities, hanging out with high-vibe friends, taking breaks from technology, and saying no to things not good for us, all contribute to raising our vibration. Activities such as drinking, abusing substances, sleeping around, masturbating to porn, overeating, under-eating, not sleeping enough, overusing technology, being under florescent lights all day long, womanizing, meaningless hook ups, spending all day and night on social media, or worse yet, on Tinder, all tend to drop our vibration. Simply put, the more we focus our attention on things that don't feel good to us, that feel ingenuine to our heart, the more we drop in vibration. The more we focus our attention on the things we love, things we enjoy, and things that make us feel good, the higher we vibe.

In any given moment, our experience of our sexuality is being influenced by our vibration and vice versa. In my study of *The Gene Keys* by Richard Rudd, I began to understand that our DNA holds within it all of the necessary components for our human evolution. However, which genes are signaled "on" and which genes are signaled "off" is very much dependent on our vibration. Thought leaders in the field of quantum physics like Dr. Joe Dispenza are already doing a masterful job of merging this ancient wisdom with scientific information, validating the influence of vibration on human physiology.

Throughout our history, our genes have had their own survival in mind. Not that long ago we lived in a much different world where life was about enduring. The immediate threat of death was everywhere. Our genes evolved to give us the best possible chance at survival. Genetically speaking, sex was a means to ensure our genes were passed on from one generation to the next. It was very much the "survival of the fittest" that Herbert Spencer suggested, the goal for males being to "spread your seed" as far and as widely as possible. To its credit, this instinct served us by creating a certain level of genetic resiliency. It drove humans to migrate and breed outside their immediate tribes and villages, in the process creating the plethora of genetic diversity that we see throughout humanity today.

We survived. We made it. We live in a much different world now than we did then. This time is inviting us to evolve again and evolve specifically our relationship to sex. Sex is so much more than just a vehicle for spreading our seed. It's more than just our primal urge to pass on our genes. Raising our vibration in regard to sex means learning how to honor sex as a sacred expression of our human potential for creativity, as well as a hallowed container for spiritual ascension. In terms of our sex energy, it means expanding our awareness to realize that whenever we have sex, masturbate, or activate our sex energy in any way, we are always conceiving and creating something. When our vibration is high because our heart is open, we create more love in the world, the greatest potential of human creativity. When our vibration is low because our heart is closed, we create more suffering, something I'm sure we're all quite familiar with.

Our vibration has a dramatic effect on what we create with our sex energy. A low vibration keeps us stuck in the shadows, living from a place of self-preservation and survival. A high vibration liberates our energy to reach for states of awareness that humans have yet to collectively access since our metaphorical "fall from grace." Just as we would never wish for a child to be conceived through the act of rape or abuse, we would also never wish to conceive with our sex energy from a place of fear, stress, frustration, greed, or anger. It's all a matter of which vibration you've hitched your wagon to—love or fear. One allows us to use our sex energy for good and the other keeps us the victim of our cognitive programming.

Remember all of those distractions we spoke about earlier? The more we transmute our sexual conditioning by raising our vibration (opening our heart), the less relevant those distractions become. Naturally, from a high vibration, we operate with a laser-like focus on our purpose and service in the world. Our heart is open to receive the guidance we need to thrive creatively and experience real intimacy in our relationships. We get to have the complete experience of sex rather than just the physical one. We get to feel the passionate ecstasy of heart orgasming bliss, as well as the healing awareness that creates love and nurtures connection. We get to have it all, a truly fulfilling sex life that not only curls our toes, but also leaves us more intimately connected with who we really are and what we're really here for.

To maintain a high vibration, it's important that we abstain from sexual activity that we know does harm. It drops our vibration and closes off our heart. It causes unnecessary suffering for everyone involved and perpetuates the conditioning we're working so hard to resolve. Even something as simple as fatigue is enough to drop our vibration and keep us from going the energetic distance in love-making, from opening to those ecstatic states of awareness. For my beloved and I, it's really an all or nothing kind of thing. We don't just have sex because we're bored or because society tells us that men and women in relationship should have sex however often in order to maintain a healthy sex life. We make love because our vibration is high and we're both feeling capable of accessing the true power of our love-making. We make love because our bodies give us a resounding "yes" to co-creating intimacy, to receiving the nourishment and connection of our union, and to offering what we create with our sex energy as a blessing for the world.

Just as our vibration matters during sex, it also matters during masturbation. When we masturbate to sexual imagery, whether in our mind or on our computer screen, objectifying a woman (whether we know them or not, whether they're our partner or not), the default way of masturbating for most men on this planet, we do so mostly in the absence of love. Again, we perpetuate the conditioning we're working so hard to resolve. When we masturbate with intention, with our full presence and conscious awareness, and with an open heart, our sex energy goes to work creating more love in the world. We'll circle back to this in later chapters, but for now you can think of it like a story once told by a Cherokee elder to his grandson. The elder said to the boy, "A fight is going on inside of me. It's a terrible fight and it's between two wolves. One is evil—he is anger, envy, sorrow, regret, greed, arrogance, self-pity, guilt, resentment, inferiority, lies, false pride, superiority, and ego." He continued, "The other is good—he is joy, peace, love, hope, serenity, humility, kindness, benevolence, empathy, generosity, truth, compassion, and faith. The same fight is going on inside of you, and inside every other person, too." The grandson thought about it for a moment and then asked his grandfather, "Which wolf will win?" To which the elder replied, "The one you feed."

Though I don't personally resonate with the word evil, this story reflects our power to choose our vibration by choosing which wolf we feed. The evil wolf is our lower-self. This is the part of us that operates unconsciously as a result of our conditioning. The good wolf is our higher-self. This is the natural part of us, who we were before our conditioning, the part of us we still are at our core, the "us" we're reclaiming by doing this work. Which wolf we feed directly impacts our vibration and whether or not we're operating as our higher-self (our pre-conditioned self) or our lower-self (our conditioned self). One makes you strong, one makes you weak. I'm not saying you have to stop having sex or stop masturbating all together. I'm simply saying don't do it unless your heart is fully open, you're operating as your higher-self, and you're holding yourself accountable to this new standard of behavioral integrity.

Doing the work to raise our vibration doesn't just impact our sex life. It positively impacts every area of our life. Something to keep in mind if you're needing an extra incentive. Vibration matters. It directly impacts what we create through sex. In a world where most men are feeding the wrong wolf, be a rebel. Feed the good wolf.

Chapter 6

A New Take on Sexual Desire

In our modern Western culture, it's generally accepted that men have some basic human needs, one of them being the need for sex. It's almost as if ejaculation has become the universally accepted key to every man's happiness. Many women I know feel pressured to have regular sex with their partner, not because they're inspired to, but because they feel they have to in order to keep their man happy. I have found that it's often the woman that bears the burden of satisfying her man's sexual desire. She's the one made responsible for his happiness. While it's important for a woman to be an invitation into intimacy, society has long validated that it's her responsibility to appease her man's sexual appetite, a nearly impossible task considering the corrupted standards set by the porn industry.

One of the many misconceptions here is that the more we have sex, the happier we will be. You may even find yourself nodding along with that statement like, "duh, yes, of course that's true." Hidden beneath this misconception is another misconception that's silently embraced by both sexes but rarely ever spoken about openly. This one says that if we're in a relationship and not sexually satisfied, it's our partner's fault, and we're justified in seeking satisfaction elsewhere. Sex, in this dynamic, becomes nothing more than an attempt to keep a man happy with the understanding that if he's not kept happy, he's liable to leave, be unfaithful, or harbor resentment. That's a lot of pressure to place on any woman, especially considering the societal expectations already placed on women to be perfect; sexy, cool, funny, athletic, etc.

Culturally, men of the West are groomed to believe that their sexual desire can only be satisfied through sex, or more specifically, through sexual acts that result in ejaculation. Western culture makes it blindingly evident that there's a direct and positive correlation between ejaculation and sexual satisfaction, where more ejaculation equates to greater satisfaction. Imprinted onto us at a young age, this cultural misconception taught us that the more we "got off," the better our lives would be. That's why it's so confusing for us when we're seemingly getting off all of the time, yet still feeling so unsatisfied inside. Most us simply conclude that we're not doing it enough, that more is the answer, further amplifying our outward search for a sense of satisfaction that can only come from within. Unfortunately, the "more rational" cannot quench the deep inner longing for satisfaction because it doesn't address the root cause. It's not a numbers game. More is not the answer. Your heart is.

On a purely primal level, we're not all that unlike most animals. We see a woman whose physicality sparks our genetic reflex and our primal instincts for procreation kick in. Our sex energy gets activated and we go out in hot pursuit, flashing our colors, doing our dance, displaying our strength, and putting on our best performance to impress our potential mate. Sounds a lot like dating, right? All of this is normal, an expression of our drive to mate and prolong our genetic existence. However, we're no longer alive to simply disperse our seed as far and as widely as possible. We're alive to reopen our hearts, join them with our sex energy, and use them both together to create our own "Heaven on Earth" reality right here and now.

For some of us, these primal forces of attraction have been wreaking havoc on our lives since the moment our sex hormones came online, thwarting our ability to channel our sex energy constructively. As a man, it's not uncommon to feel sexually attracted to several different women throughout the course of a single day. In this world full of beautiful people, all we need to do is step outside and inevitably we'll encounter someone that excites us in this way. Are we bad for feeling this? Are we wrong for feeling an in the moment attraction towards a woman? Should we feel shameful? The simple answer is, no.

It's natural for men to feel attracted to women, and to other men. These forces have long been the foundation for procreation, which isn't something to shame considering it's how we all got here. It's only when our conditioned mind gets ahold of this excitement that we create problems. When greeted from the perspective of our high vibration that I shared about in the previous chapter, our sexual desire actually has nothing to do with the other person whatsoever. Yes, that is what I just said. It has to do with us, not them. Our sexual desire is our higher-self, that highest "vibing" part of us, being reflected back to us through the vehicle of another. You can think of it as an in-the-moment communication from your higher-self to your everyday-self saying, "Hey, it's me, your higher-self, the one responsible for guiding you through life. Did you forget about me? Breathe, circulate this energy throughout your body, and raise your in-the-moment vibration. It's a gift for you to feel such heightened sensations, put them to good use."

Yes, I just said higher-self and sex in the same sentence. Again, here is what I mean when I say higher-self. There is a part of us that can only be satisfied by deeply knowing and receiving who we are at our source, and who we are at our source is not our body, our mind, or the name we were given at birth. It's not our personality, our habits and behaviors, or the career path we've chosen. It's an energy that, when present, illuminates our body with life. Anyone that's ever been to a funeral home and looked inside a casket can attest to this. We see it when we look into each other's eyes. We see it in ourselves when we stand in front of the mirror and look into our own eyes. Some call this our spirit, some call it our soul. I call this part of us our higher-self, but you can call it by whatever name feels right for you.

No matter what you call it, we all yearn to merge and unite

with this aspect of ourselves. It's what sends us on our spiritual journey to begin with. In life we're often tricked into believing that more of something outside of us is the answer to satisfying this inner yearning, but that's simply not the case. Most of us spend years, some entire lifetimes, seeking to fill this desire for our higher-self through external means. Sex, for men, is one of the most common means we use to try to fill this desire, but it never works. It can never work because it will never be enough to satisfy the intensity of our yearning to merge with who we really are at our source. Trust me, I've tried.

Yes, as crazy as it might sound, I want you to relate to your sexual desire as a direct communication from your higher-self. Why? Because it the most honest thing we can do. Believe it or not, it's actually dishonest for us to feel sexual desire towards another human being and pretend it's only our primal instinct to "disperse our seed." We're especially dishonest with ourselves anytime we tangle our sexual desire with our cognitive conditioning, never acknowledging it in its totality. When we deny our sexual desire of its true nature, we deny ourselves of receiving our higher-self, the only experience that ever truly fulfills our inner yearning.

There's a huge difference between tuning in to our higher-self and sexually objectifying someone. One leads us to connect with a part of us that we long for and the other harms the innocence of another. Unfortunately, 99 times out of 100 we mistakenly make this experience about the other person; "Damn she's fine. Phew, look at that body. Mmm, the things I would do." While it's appropriate to appreciate the beauty of others, it's inappropriate for us to put our sex energy onto others without their consent. Sexual desire is a beautiful thing when it's worked with consciously, but when it's channeled unconsciously, it can cause men to project their sex energy onto women who they believe are the source of their desire.

Again, it's not the woman we desire. It's the experience of

merging with our higher-self that we desire. Think about it, your sexual desire is an aspect of you. You're the one feeling it inside your body. It's emanating from inside you, not entering into you from an external source. How could it possibly have anything to do with anyone else? You think it's desire *for* something, or more specifically, for someone, when really it just *is*. When the desire is misplaced, women can easily become the victims. We discussed this earlier. It seems harmless, but it's not. You can think of this as a form of energetic groping. If it were happening physically, there would be legal consequences, but because it's happening energetically, it's tolerated.

Sometimes this can temporarily validate a woman for her physical appearance, giving her a short-term boost of energy and the opportunity to take advantage of this exchange. The danger is that it allows society to overly sexualize women, so that using sex energy and sex appeal becomes a means to manipulate others and get ahead. Don't get me wrong, this absolutely goes both ways. Sexual manipulation is used by both sexes, but for woman, this behavior is usually an adopted technique because our culture told her that her survival depended on it. It's not uncommon for a woman being energetically groped to feel abruptly exposed or unsafe. If she does become aware of the source of her discomfort, the man projecting his sex energy onto her, there's often not much she can do about it other than remove herself from the situation as soon as she can. All of this is considered "normal" from a cultural perspective because the culture itself tolerates men being unconscious with their sex energy. Culture is nothing more than the accepted way of doing things among a group of people. It's not static. It can be changed.

Let me re-emphasize this here, any time we feel sexual desire towards another human being, what we're actually feeling is our higher-self attempting to get our attention. Our higher-self is saying things like, "Hey (fill in your name here), remember me, your higher-self? I'm up here. Raise your vibration so that you and I can hang out together." Why would our higher-self care to use sexual desire as its means to communicate such things to us? Because think about it, as a man, what seizes your awareness more than sex? Our higher-self desires our attention so it can deliver to us guidance, insights, ideas, inspirations, and intuitive nudges that are one hundred percent in alignment with our life purpose. They want us to be close to them so that they can direct us through life, making sure we don't miss out on what we're actually here for. Our in-the-moment vibration absolutely impacts our ability to receive guidance from our higher-self. If our vibe is low, we'll go about pursuing our low frequency sexual desire while missing the bigger picture, projecting our sex energy out onto others and getting caught up in our own personal melodrama. If our vibe is high, we either won't experience this lower frequency sexual desire at all, or, when we do, we'll immediately recognize it for what it is, breathe, and tune in to the energy of our higher-self.

Wondering how that can be so? Well, for one, our higher-self is brilliant. It knows that sexual desire is a powerful primal energy. When partnered with our awareness and breath, it's powerful enough to lift us closer to our higher-self. When channeled this way, our sexual desire becomes a spark, a conscious reminder for us to circulate our sex energy up into our heart and receive our higher-self, an experience often described with words like euphoria, ecstasy, elation, and bliss. It's all a matter of vibration. At the lowest vibration, we relate to each other as sex objects and use each other to "get off." At this higher vibration, we mirror back to one another the ecstatic energy of our higher-selves. Approached from this perspective, we can actually see how brilliant a setup it all really is, completely rigged in our favor.

Sexual desire is also an element of novelty. When something is new it's exciting to the senses, that's just basic human chemistry. Yes, I'm talking about the honeymoon phase and the excitement around meeting someone new, when the sex is frequent and seemingly all that matters. The more time we spend with someone, the more the regularity of our love-making naturally relaxes. Some experts say this is a bad thing, something to avoid at all costs, the sign of a dying relationship. I say, this is completely normal, the way it's meant to be. The more time we spend in relationship, the more our love and the way we express it naturally matures. The intensity of the love-making is still exhilarating, it simply makes room for other things that are equally as satisfying.

A man's conditioning can keep him from maturing in this way. If we're still watching porn or something of the like, our sexual desire is barred from maturing. We're likely to be trapped by our boyish desire, placing too much attention on "getting off" and not enough attention on the quality of our everyday life, on connecting with our higher-self. This not only keeps us from receiving our higher-self, but also keeps us from tending to the other areas of life where we could be drawing deep satisfaction. Our brain gets tricked into looking for newness, something exciting outside of the norm, all the while missing out on the grand adventure of being fully present with the woman right here in front of us. Novelty is exciting, but that's all it really is. It lacks the depth that cultivates true satisfaction.

I'm sure by now you're probably wondering how to take this primal evolutionary force called "spread your seed" and convert it into your most profound means for expanded awareness. I'm sure you're also probably wondering how to navigate the old patterning, cultural imprinting, and early-life conditioning that has us ceaselessly seeking to fulfill our sexual desire through external means. First things first. This conversation in particular is more about awareness than it is anything else. The first means of transmuting our superficial sexual desire into its higher purpose is to be radically honest and accepting of its presence.

The more we try to hide from it the stronger it becomes.

There's no escaping our sexual desire because we're not meant to. Instead, we're meant to accept, understand, evolve, and receive it fully, by moving towards it rather than away. When we attempt to suppress our sexual desire (and many of us do) by burying it down inside of us, we inherently reject a part of ourselves only to have it resurface one hundred-fold later down the road. This is our shame at work, and eventually leads to a distorted expression of our sexuality. We focus so much energy on keeping the desire at bay that there's very little energy left over for self-expression. What we resist persists. When we pursue our every desire attempting to exhaust it, we quickly discover its inexhaustible nature. In this scenario, we end up quickly depleting ourselves of our creative life force, and again, we're left with little energy left over.

Secondly, it's important for us to stay in the role of the observer. We are not wrong for having assumed the conditioning that was given to us, but we are responsible for managing it differently. Being the observer provides us with just enough internal spaciousness to witness this pure primal force getting mixed up with our porn conditioning. As the observer, we can have compassion for ourselves without making it mean anything about who we are morally. This primal force that has seemingly dominated our awareness since puberty is actually quite impersonal to us. Everyone in the world has it, and nearly everyone in the world has it tangled up with their conditioning. There is nothing wrong with us. Only a program put somewhere that it doesn't belong. With awareness, we can remove it, or at least remove its power over us.

Though this primal force is impersonal to us, our sensitivity to it is not. The same sensitivity that initially caused us to feel overwhelmed by our sexual energy now provides us with a profound awareness of its presence, helping us to do this work. We were created sensitive to this energy because we were always meant to work with it in a powerful way. It's one of the most important reasons why we're here, to heal the misuse of sex energy and use it for good this time around. So next time you're out in the world and you come across someone who ignites this force within you, become aware of it. Don't feed it, and don't blame yourself for having it, just observe and breathe consciously. With enough practice, you'll become grateful for the reminders to connect with your higher-self.

It's good to note here again that his whole process of transmuting our sexual desire into its higher purpose requires honesty and acceptance. Without our full awareness and acceptance of our sexual desire, we are doomed to fall into the same cycle of pursuing our desire outwardly while feeling unsatisfied and shameful inwardly. The bigger picture is that all of this is very much rigged in our favor. It takes practice and an eventual mastery of this awareness to go beyond the current limitations of our conditioning, but when we know better, we do better. At some point, we'll have to come to terms with what a powerful force for good our sex energy can be and choose to direct it towards creating something meaningful.

It's really not that hard either. It just takes a little bit of intention and some consistent practice. For now, just remember that when you find yourself attracted to someone else, you are really having a part of you that you long to connect with, your higher-self, mirrored back to you. As we eliminate our outer distractions and start to recognize our desire for what it is, we'll naturally come to embody our sex energy. We'll stop making it about other people and realize this is a part of *us* that we're meant to interact with consciously. That means we'll stop wasting "our seed" and instead use it to give life to all of those things that actually have meaning to us. If it's not clear to you by now, then let's make it clear once and for all. This is about you, your journey, your growth, and making your life and the world around you better.

It's time for us to let go of our incessant attempts to fulfill our superficial desire through sex. It's time for us to orient ourselves around the truth. Our superficial sexual desire will always come and go based on our vibration, but our desire to merge with our higher-self will remain forever. "Heaven on Earth" is when we choose to merge. It may seem too good to be true, but it's not. You'll just have to merge and find out for yourself.

Chapter 7

The Father Wound

Born into the heart of every little boy are some of the most daunting questions he'll ever have to answer in his lifetime. Questions like, "Am I really good enough? Do I really have what it takes? Am I really a man?" Sensitive by our very nature, these questions live in some of the most tender places within a boy's heart. Their presence is no mistake, these questions propel us out into the world on a mission to discover their answers. Typically surfacing around the age of puberty, a time that marks a boy's physical maturation into manhood, the answers to these questions define our masculine identity; the masculine framework through which we see, perceive, and experience the world, and ourselves in it. The result of this process becomes who we know ourselves to be, from the inside out, as a man. Once defined, our masculine identity travels with us throughout our entire life as our benchmark or reference point for who we are as a man. It becomes the masculine filter through which we see, perceive, and interact with the world.

Every man was once a boy and every boy, at one time or another, saw his father through the eyes of his innocence. As children, we often associate the word "dad" with other words like superhero, hero, champion, idol, and god. When we were young, our fathers meant the world to us. We admired them, even worshiped them at times. They could do no wrong. They had the Midas touch. We wanted nothing more than to be by their side, win their affection, and make them proud. When our questions about our masculine identity initially surfaced, we naturally turned to our father for answers. Hidden behind every conversation and every interaction were the questions, "Dad, am I really a man? Do I really have what it takes to be a man? Am I really equipped for the job?" Whether they were aware of it or not, our father's answers to these silent questions absolutely impacted the construction of our masculine identity. Our father's answers determined whether or not we saw ourselves as a man as we entered into adulthood.

For most of us, the answers we received from our father to the questions above were insufficient at best. Having not been told, "Yes, you are a man. Yes, you have what it takes. Yes, you are more than enough," we entered into adulthood and the complexities of the modern world still longing for answers. Sometimes we did get answers, just not the kind that any boy wants to hear, our fathers the recipients of their own wounding. Not having heard what we needed to hear from our childhood hero, we sought our answers elsewhere.

Many of us turned to our career, learned how to make a lot of money, and let our wealth buffer our insecurities around being a man. Others of us took to aggression, learned how to pick fights, and found ourselves constantly battling other men to prove our strength. Still, others of us tried to numb our pain, turning to substances that we thought would help us forget the past, as well as how we felt about it. For those of us that could not find our answers amongst the men in our lives, we turned to women. We unconsciously sexualized our father wound and sought validation for our masculine identity through women and sex. Sex, and our underlying sexuality, became our modus operandi for proving our manliness, a burden that sex was never meant to carry.

My father was and remains a very loving man. He's a baby boomer, born from a generation of men that were taught to be strong, not cry, toughen up, and work hard. The first born child in a succession of eight, my father was held responsible for assisting in the rearing of his siblings. He was expected to set a good example for his brothers and sisters to follow. Back then, men weren't taught the value of sharing themselves vulnerably.

Having been raised in a pretty tough manner by my grandfather, my dad learned early on that emotions meant weakness, that real men don't cry.

He adapted by showing his love in other ways, primarily through acts of service. He was always the provider, a man that would work until his fingers bled to take care of his family. Rarely did I ever see him rest. He was often the first one up in the morning and the last one to hit the pillow at night. Occasionally, as he aged, he would pass out on the living room sofa chair, briefly revealing his utter exhaustion. He'd mow the lawn, cook dinner, do the grocery shopping, fix our cars, pull weeds, clean the pool, return the recyclables, and reliably work on any ongoing DIY home project to keep our home healthy. Occasionally, there would be a home project that was too big for him to handle on his own, in which case I, being his only son, was enlisted for the job. Even though I initially resisted the thought of re-shingling the roof or power washing the back patio, I was always happy to pitch in a helping hand.

When my dad wasn't taking care of his to-do list, he was often supporting us kids with our own endeavors, like sports, for instance. My father helped coach nearly all of my sports teams right up until the day I reached high school. He was dedicated too, always giving it his all. He spent countless hours throughout my youth hitting ground balls, throwing fast balls, teaching me how to box out, pivot, shoot free throws, block, and throw a spiral. He never missed a game, at least not any that I can remember. In the spring it was baseball, football in the late summer and fall, and basketball in the winter. Year round my father showed up and cheered me on, as well as all of the other boys that were a part of my sports teams.

Beyond sports, my father also loved the outdoors. My sisters and I were lucky enough to spend much of our youth at our family cabin in Northern Michigan. There it was all nature, wildlife, adventure, and play. The woods were our playground and the lakes our swimming pools. My father took me hunting, fishing, boating, camping, hiking, and on many other adventures in the wild. He showed me how to shoot a gun, how to use a pocketknife, how to clean a fish, and how to skin a deer. I'll never forget the two of us sitting there together in the dead of winter in our deer blind, smack dab in the middle of my grandfather's sixty acres of swampland, freezing our asses off waiting for deer. I'm sure they could hear my teeth chattering from a mile away. Present to my predicament, my dad leaned in and quietly asked, "Pst, are you cold?" Blue-faced and shivering uncontrollably, I quickly replied, "no," not wanting to seem like a baby.

It's probably hard to imagine that I could have gotten stuck with anything "negative" from my childhood, especially as it relates to my father. However, my father, like all men, had his own shortcomings. While he inherited a great and many valuable qualities from the generation before him: hard work, perseverance, commitment, dedication, loyalty, and grit, what he didn't learn from my grandparents was how to translate his emotions into words. He didn't know how to share his feelings. As a child and young man, I naturally received love through physical touch, quality time, and words of affirmation. The quality time piece he nailed, but as I matured, I longed for his words. A carpenter by trade, my father could talk all day long about what he was building at work or how he managed to fix the downstairs furnace. That was easy for him. What wasn't so easy was looking me in my eyes and telling me he loved me or taking a moment to share with me that he was proud.

As I aged and began navigating those more challenging life experiences like puberty and the onset of my sex energy, I felt like I didn't have anyone I could talk to. When my questions of whether or not I had what it took to be a man were at their peak, my father's shortcomings around verbally expressing his heart had an impact on me. John Eldridge, in his book *Wild at*

Heart, suggests that masculinity bestows masculinity. In other words, the father (or the father figure) bestows (conveys as a gift) masculinity to his son. Not that mothers don't have an enormous role in cultivating masculinity; they absolutely do, but by design, or by default you could say, there is a part of every man that can only be filled by the masculinity passed on to him by his father.

I longed to know, in my heart of hearts, that my father saw me as man. I wanted to feel that, no matter what concerns, fears, or worries I had about life, love, sex, and whatever else might lie beyond boyhood, in my father's eyes, I absolutely had everything it took to carve out my own path and be a man in the world. That knowing, for all men, must come from their father (or the masculine role model acting as father). Without this knowing, boys inevitably wander out into the very complex ways of the modern world looking for evidence of their masculinity, usually in all the wrong places. This is the father wound.

I wandered into my high school years still questioning my masculinity and looking for opportunities to prove that I was a man. I became highly competitive towards other men in everything from sports and academics to keg stands and drinking contests. I strove to be the best at everything I did, because for me, my masculine identity was on the line. I did everything I could to look more manly. I lifted weights, shaved my head, drank beer, played my music way too loud, and had a lot of girlfriends. I thought that if I played the part right, at least my friends would see me as a man. Maybe then I'd finally believe it for myself.

I still remember a senior from my high school making fun of me on my first day of weightlifting class. I was bench pressing when he approached, three years ahead of me in physical maturity. He looked over at me, pointed, laughed, and said out loud in front of everyone in the gym, "what's that, your max?"

As in, is that all you can bench press? Unfortunately for me, it was. Yes, I was maxing out at 135 pounds as a freshman in high school, which felt incredibly vulnerable to me at the time, but there were a lot of things that felt vulnerable back then; like being a virgin, having zero facial hair, and virtually no muscle mass.

Point being, any time I encountered another guy that seemed like a manly man to me, you know, "muscles, money, and mojo," my masculine identity felt threatened. Feeling so uncomfortable around men and having yet to receive any real answers from the masculine role models in my life, I naturally gravitated towards women. I started seeking validation for my masculinity through the women I interacted with, especially sexually. I unknowingly sexualized my father wound and began investing my time and energy into becoming a sexual dynamo. From my perspective, sexual prowess was one of the key factors for measuring manliness, and one that obviously didn't require me to be around other men.

My promiscuity developed, at least in part, as a way for me to answer my own questions about being a man. Every time I slept with a woman and succeeded in leaving her satisfied, it validated my masculinity. Every time word got out about my performance and the rumors made their way around to the others guys my age, I was further validated. The catch-22 was that the opposite was also true. Every time I fooled around with a girl and failed at delivering her an earth shattering experience; every time I missed the mark, got burnt out on trying so hard, or was too intoxicated to perform, it diminished my masculine identity.

As I'm sure you can imagine, a lot was weighing on my sexual performance. I wasn't stepping into the sex space with an open heart or with the intention of creating intimacy. I was stepping into sex to prove I was a man. Unfortunately, all of the power that I imagined I had, the power to pleasure a woman and prove my manliness, was actually power I was giving away every time I had sex. When she enjoyed herself and spread good rumors about me, I got to walk confidently as a man. When she didn't enjoy herself, had an okay time, or got upset with how things unfolded after the fact, the rumors that spread were debilitating.

Relationships somewhat lifted this incessant need to perform. Getting to know someone on more than just a superficial level certainly helped me relax some of my performance anxiety. By this time, I had become what you could consider a seasoned lover, but my sense of masculinity still remained in the hands of my partner. Only instead of being strangers, now the women I dated were even closer to my heart and loaded with more ammunition. Now it wasn't just my sexual performance that was defining me as a man, but also my performance as a partner.

When my girlfriend was happy, I was winning at being a man. Whenever she was unhappy, for me, it was because I was somehow failing at being "the man" in the relationship. I told myself, if I was different, then she'd be happy. It was all very personal to me because, again, my internal sense of masculinity was on the line. I gave my partner the power to make me feel like Alexander the Great in one moment and a heaping pile of shit in the next. My desire to feel like a man, to answer the unanswered questions in my heart, were leading me to seek validation for my masculinity outside of myself; an unhealthy pressure to place on any romantic relationship, let alone on sex.

When relationships didn't work, pornography usually did. Here was a space where my mind could play out any sexual fantasy without the risk of failure. In terms of my performance, each visit the female performers would be reliably left wildly intoxicated by me, virtually validating through fantasy my sense of masculinity. With an endless supply of novelty, I was never short of a woman that would sexually worship me as god. Of course, none of it was real, but my mind didn't necessarily care about that. I was coping, but just as my promiscuity wasn't enough to keep my father wound at bay, pornography wasn't either.

My sense of having satisfied my need for validation continuously lasted for shorter and shorter periods of time, meaning my visits became more and more frequent. I had no idea that I was looking to porn, sex, and my romantic relationships to validate my masculine identity. I just thought I was going about it how everyone else did. In fact, I don't think I thought about it at all until years later, when I finally paused long enough to question why all of my romantic relationships had failed, why I had such an unhealthy reliance on porn, and why I was wasting so much time and energy chasing sexual encounters that never amounted to anything meaningful.

The only way out of sexualizing my father wound and over-sexualizing myself to prove I was a match to our culture's depiction of "manly," was to acknowledge that I was using sex and my sexual relationships with women to validate my masculinity. It didn't have to manifest as sleeping around or being promiscuous either. I had built an obsessive relationship with porn because it was a space where I could cope with my wounding without ever having to address it. Regardless of how this wound becomes sexualized, the key is to see it for what it is. Every "player" was once a little boy that didn't hear what he needed to from his father. He wasn't properly bestowed masculinity, at least not the authentic kind, so he attempted to conquer it through women and sex. He became promiscuous, whether virtually or in reality, to conquer his desire to feel like a man.

Seeing it for what it is lifts the illusion and allows us to take responsibility for ourselves as men. Rather than living into fantasy, we're given the opportunity to understand what it is we're meant to learn by turning inward and facing our wound directly. Ironically, this just so happens to be our authentic initiation into manhood. Truth is, we initiate ourselves into manhood through learning what we're meant to learn from our life experiences and embodying those lessons. When we look deeper into our life experiences, we see that we're already provided with every situation we need to fully embody our authentic masculine expression. The issue is that we spend most of our time trying to avoid our wounding, afraid to feel the pain, and miss out on the masculine initiations we so desperately desire. When we see our wounding for what it is and choose to lean into it rather than away, we say "yes" to the initiation that inevitably results in our authentic masculine embodiment. In terms of sex, we learn to relate to love-making as a gift that an embodied man and an embodied woman share together, rather than an experience that a man needs in order to feel like a man.

But how do we get there from here? How do we get to the place where our authentic masculine flows naturally through our sexuality? We have to go back to go forwards. We have to go back to our young life and reexamine our early relationship with our father. We have to look and ask ourselves the tough questions like, "did I really receive what I needed? Did I hear what I needed to hear? What was I left with, for better or for worse? How have I sexualized my wound?" Asking these questions and examining their answers allows us to embody the lessons we came here to learn. It allows the wound to serve its purpose. Once we stare into the heart of our father wound, feel it, process it, and let it go, it releases its grip on us. Stripped of our wounding, sex becomes what it was always meant to be, a natural and sacred expression of our humanity. Engaging in love-making from this place of wholeness opens us to further receive the true power of heart centered love-making, including the intimacy created from it. We also heal our masculine bloodline, ensuring that these wounds do not get passed on from our generation to the next.

When I learned that I was using sex to validate my masculine identity, everything changed. It was a light bulb moment. Suddenly everything inauthentic about my sexuality was illuminated. In that moment, I realized that most of my sexual experiences up until that point in my life had not been an authentic reflection of me, or at least not the man I was committed to being. It made sense that I had felt so helplessly trapped by my sexual desire, my need to perform, and so unfulfilled by my sexual experiences, because I had unconsciously enlisted sex to protect me from feeling the pain of my wounding. I had placed a huge burden on sex and my relationships with women to distract me from feeling my father wound. This awakening not only allowed me to forgive myself and my father, but also allowed me to address the young man inside of me that just wanted to feel seen by his father. I was able to talk to him, have compassion for his life experience, and remind him with my words of what he had been wanting to hear all along; that he was indeed a man, a good man at that, someone that I was extremely proud of.

My quest to prove myself as a man came to end when I paused long enough to evaluate all the ways in which life had already initiated me into manhood. What I had been so desperately seeking was already right here inside of me all along. I had just been searching for it outside of myself, rather than the one place it could actually be found. I realized that I didn't receive the traditional bestowing of masculinity because I wasn't meant to, because I came here to do masculinity differently. I also realized that masculinity is inherently undefinable because we as men are meant to define it for ourselves, in a way that's authentic to us. That means there are as many expressions of masculinity as there are men on this planet. The important thing is to discover which of those expressions are most authentic to you, even if they don't conform to the norm.

I've stopped putting so much pressure on sex to make me feel like a man and started allowing it to be a celebration of the intimacy and connection already present within my romantic relationship. I feel better capable of being around women without needing to sexualize them in any way, without needing their validation, without needing anything from them at all. In a sense, you could say that I was able to take a big step forward in healing my relationship with women by directly facing my father wound.

The opportunity here is to bring an aspect of our masculinity into greater wholeness by consciously revisiting and healing our father wound. All wounds are healed through love. This doesn't mean blaming our father or the generation that preceded us for how we feel. That being said, anger, rage, heartbreak, sadness, and disappointment all have their place along the healing journey. Honor whatever surfaces for you as you revisit your father wound, but also be mindful not to project your suffering onto others. The more you can be honest with your feelings and what remains in your heart regarding your relationship with your father, the better off you're going to be. This wound can be especially charged with emotion. Be responsible for that emotion while still fully honoring it. When all else fails, come back to your center. Breathe into your emotion and give it space to surface. Don't push it away or stuff it back down. It's wanting to be loved and accepted by you.

Chapter 8

Restoring Our Inner Innocence

Simply put, most of us did not receive the early life environment we needed to feel fully safe to fly. Born into this world little sponges, we quickly absorbed our environment's relationship to things like sex, money, love, family, faith, work, etc. Our parents were our greatest influence. Chances are they parented us the same way they were parented, which is precisely how wounds like the father wound get passed down from one generation to the next. What's important to remember here, especially in the context of this conversation, is that we're never the victims of our parents' conditioning.

At the highest level, we choose our parents for the precise life experience we'll have with them as our parents. These are the pre-life agreements we make with other souls then forget about once we're born. On a soul level, it's quite honorable that our parents signed up to be a source of contrast for us, one that inevitably propelled us onto our spiritual path. Regardless of what our relationship with them looks like now, we can honor our parents for their essential role in our lives, knowing they did the best they could with the tools they were given, wounding and all.

Many of us had early life experiences that impacted us in big ways, sometimes seemingly for the worst. Maybe it was a divorce, the death of a loved one, sexual abuse, physical or emotional abuse, or the feeling of being entirely repressed, like we had no voice, forced to fit into a box we hated. When the impactful event initially happened, no one sat us down to help us process it. When we were young, it was common for events to happen without any explanation for them whatsoever. Our parents and the other adults in our lives thought they were protecting us by not talking about it. In reality, this only left our emotions regarding the experience entirely unaddressed. Those emotions still live inside of us. For better or for worse, our young life experiences are impacting us today just as much as they did the day that they happened.

Only in the last few years have I been revisiting these early life experiences with the intention of understanding how I was genuinely impacted by them. I wanted to comprehend how they had molded me, what part they played in the formation of my identity, my personality, my ways of being, my emotional expression, and my thought patterns. For example, because of the emotionally repressed environment I grew up in, I was very good at suppressing my emotions. I rarely ever cried, but also rarely ever let myself feel joy and excitement. I got good at playing the middle road, not too emotionally high and not too emotionally low. On the inside, this left me feeling pretty disconnected from life, but on the outside it had me appear "really put together."

It just so happens that one of the few nicknames that stuck throughout my early adulthood was "Mr. Perfect." I came from a good family, was fairly successful, intelligent, attractive, athletic, no emotional baggage, or at least that's the way it seemed from the outside looking in. Anyone that got too close to me eventually felt the wrath of my unexpressed emotions coming out as anger. I was mad. Even as a child I remember getting upset, holding my breath, clenching my muscles, and pushing all the blood in my body up into my face, turning it red and making my veins pop out. I was genuinely angry, but for the rest of my family, this was just a form of free entertainment.

Sure, it was cute then, but now as an adult, not so much. As an adult, anger looked like me verbally lashing out at my romantic partners, conveying everything that bothered me about them in one aggressive blow. Not the healthiest form of emotional expression. Certainly not the most constructive either. My episodes of anger had a huge impact on all of my romantic relationships. It seemed unavoidable. The first three to six months would pass without any real issues, but that was my limit for emotional repression. The little things I'd left unexpressed would build up. Overwhelmed by what I felt inside, I'd unleash it all in the form of verbal daggers, doing lethal damage to the relationship, and leaving my romantic partners incredibly confused and hurt. "Why does it feel like this person that says he loves me, actually hates me?"

Romantic relationships can be a profound mirror for the unresolved emotional pain of our past. In other words, all the things I hadn't yet emotionally resolved about the events of my childhood, especially in relation to my mother and father, were now showing up in my romantic relationships to be acknowledged, processed, resolved, and healed. It took me quite a while to get this, but when I did, I realized what an asshole I had been. I was caught in this unhealthy cycle of blaming my romantic partners for the way I felt inside rather than seizing these upsets as my opportunity to intentionally explore the honest source of my pain.

What I learned from these experiences and others similar to them are now some of the most potent tools in my toolbox, the most important by far being inner child work. That is, maintaining a strong, healthy, and constructive relationship with my inner child. Each one of us lives with our four-, five-, or six-year-old self still alive inside of us. No, I don't mean literally, of course, but metaphorically. Or better yet, energetically. This is the part of us that never grew up. It's our inner innocence, that part of us that views life with a childlike wonder, playful enthusiasm, and an exuberant spirit. It's the part of us that remains in Neverland as we age and take on our adult responsibilities. It's also the part of us that can sabotage our romantic relationships or have us show up as Peter Pan in the bedroom, running from our shadow, behaving like one of the lost boys.

Our inner child has been with us throughout all of our adult experiences, including our sexual experiences. He still maintains the same perspective on life that he had when we were a kid and has been responding to our life experiences through our adult body. Have you ever seen an adult throw a temper tantrum? That's their inner child at play. By becoming aware of our inner child we can not only heal the pain of our childhood, the same pain that's still impacting us today, but we can also develop into better lovers, and certainly, better partners.

Rather than acting from our childhood wounds, we can recognize the difference between our inner child and us, address our inner child's needs directly, and prevent ourselves from projecting our childhood pain onto our partner. This is how we restore our inner innocence. Healing our inner innocence liberates the energy of play in our relationships, but also allows us to show up as men instead of boys. It helps us mature our boyhood relationship to sex by differentiating our inner child from the man inside of us. In terms of sex, we get to have it all; passion and playfulness, intimacy and fun, depth and lightheartedness, without the same boyhood immaturity, without our unresolved childhood pain thwarting our attempts at intimacy.

Instead of the old masculine model, kill the boy and let the man be born, this version includes love. I say, heal the boy and the man will emerge. Heal the boy and bring the best of him, his purity, his tenderness, and his joy, into adulthood. When we're aware of our inner child, we're better able to hear him, listen to him, understand him, talk with him, be there for him, and help him feel safe. Ultimately, we're able to reparent him in all the ways that he needed to be parented back when we were him. This allows us to mature into the adults we are now, rather than live from the wounding of our childhood. It's not that this child is bad in any way. It's actually quite the opposite. Our inner child is extraordinary. He's creative, playful, joyous, imaginative, and energetic. He's just not meant to be running the show. I know, it's a strange thing to consider, especially if you've never been introduced to inner child work before.

"Wait. So, you're telling me I have a little boy inside of me, my childhood-self, that's everyday interacting with the world around me through my physical body?" I am one hundred percent confirming that is absolutely the case. I am also offering that it's our inner child that's responding to the events in our adult lives, especially in our romantic relationships, through the lens of what we felt and never emotionally processed as children. It's actually our inner child that can feel so hurt and scared in response to our everyday adult interactions, not the man in us. Whenever our inner child does feel hurt, we react with anger, unknowingly trying to protect him from feeling the pain.

Anger is our unconscious way of protecting our inner child from re-experiencing the emotional pain we felt as children. As adults, we lash out in anger not because we're being dealt a fresh wound, but because an interaction we're having is reminding us of an old wound, an emotional pain that we felt initially during childhood. The hurt simply never got resolved and we've been living with it inside of us ever since. By resolved, I don't mean fixed… I mean acknowledged, felt, accepted, and healed. When our unresolved hurt is triggered in our romantic relationships, it puts us into a fight, flight, or freeze response, meaning fight (anger) is not our only option. Sometimes we run from the pain, sometimes we're paralyzed by it. Other times we shut down.

We've all witnessed children screaming bloody murder in one moment only to be laughing and giggling the next. This is because children are masterful at feeling an emotion and simply letting it out. Because they have no filter and hold nothing back, no emotional energy gets trapped inside their bodies. They feel it, they express it. Period, end of story. That is, until they learn what's acceptable and what's not acceptable to emotionally express from the adults in their lives. Then the suppression begins. By the time we arrive to adulthood, we typically have decades worth of unexpressed emotional energy trapped inside our body, most of which is being held onto by our inner child. It's not even a question of if, but what and where. What emotions are we still holding onto from our childhood and where are they being stored in our body?

A quick little story of how this relates. I first discovered my inner child all the way back in September of 2017, when Makenzie and I were traveling through Guatemala for some work and play. We thought the two would mingle seamlessly. They did not. Makenzie had some unexpected and pressing work pop up that threw me off my game. Each day she was worked well past our agreed upon stop time and I had no idea how to predict how much work she actually had. Each day I worked up until our agreed upon stop time, then twiddled my thumbs waiting for her to finish.

Not wanting to impose more stress onto an already stressful situation, I withheld requesting a new stop time, but my frustration was clearly building. My tone with Makenzie changed to reflect my frustration, but I still tried to keep my cool. I was caught in a state of limbo. On one side I desired to be there for her during this clearly stressful time. I wanted to nourish her and reassure her that she wasn't in this alone. On the other side, I felt jaded because the adventure that I thought we had come here to have was quickly getting sacrificed for the work that needed to be done.

I felt hurt, but it was a familiar hurt. You know the disappointment you feel when you make plans with someone you love and they cancel on you last minute, or better yet, don't show up at all. You're there waiting for them constantly checking the clock. The excitement I felt in anticipation of our adventure quickly turned into feelings of rejection, because to me, it seemed that work was more important than the time we had planned to spend together. I felt hurt, but instead of sharing honestly, I projected my hurt outward as frustration. I started shutting down, unconsciously closing off my heart to protect myself from feeling rejected, which left my expressions towards Makenzie rather cold and heartless.

This whole situation, however, was reflecting something much deeper and closer to my core. I was the youngest of three children. As a kid, both of my parents worked full-time. When they weren't working, they were often doing other things like mowing the lawn, preparing dinner, doing yardwork, or some other practical to-do list item that adults do to take care of themselves and their families. I remember many times as a kid asking my parents, especially my father, to come outside and play with me in the yard. When they would say "no," because of whatever other work they needed to do, I would feel personally rejected. To me, it felt like my parents had other things in life that they valued more than me. In those moments, I didn't feel like the most important thing in their lives, even though I really wanted to.

When they would say no, many times without an explanation, my little mind would assume all kinds of things. "They don't *really* love me. I'm not as important to them as they say I am. They don't want to be around me. I'm better off just playing by myself." All the same assumptions that I was now making with Makenzie in Guatemala. My inner child felt rejected, hurt, unimportant, and uncherished. Anytime I felt that way as a child, I would go off and play by myself, each time closing my heart a little more towards my parents. Now, as my adult-self in Guatemala, my inner child was again wanting to go off and play by himself, all because he didn't feel like a priority to his best friend. He started closing down his heart, not wanting to feel the pain of rejection. My inner child was reacting to this situation based on what I had felt in similar situations as a child, things that I had yet to go back and properly process with him as an adult.

After a few bouts of anger expressed as verbal lashings, me trying to protect my innocence from the pain he was feeling, I finally got the memo. My inner child was asking *me* to be there for him, wanting *me* to see and acknowledge his hurt, wanting *me* to reassure him that no matter what, he's always a priority to me. He was wanting me to soothe his pain, and he was throwing a temper tantrum inside of my adult body to get my attention. It was a massive lesson for me in seeing the value of having a working relationship with my inner child; to be able to connect with him, listen to him, understand him, and be present with him not only in moments when he's hurting, but also in moments when he's delighted too. My inner child was asking for me to be present with his feelings, and for the first time in my life, I was listening.

Our inner child needs reparenting. He needs to know that he's once again safe to feel and express his emotions, no matter what they might be. He needs a parent that will listen, understand, and encourage him to share what he's feeling. We are those parents now. We are the ones that must turn inward, re-establish a relationship with our inner child, and love that child in all the ways he needed to feel loved back when we were him. We are the ones that must embrace his sensitivity, his empathic nature, his innocent heart, and his emotional expression. It's up to us to share with our inner child all of the things that he needed to hear when we were him; things like, it's okay to feel sad, it's not your fault your parents are upset right now, you didn't do anything wrong, you're safe to go and play. Whatever it is he desired to hear in his moments of need, we're the ones to express that to him now.

Why? Because we can. Because we have the capacity for that level of sensitivity towards our inner child, and because it's necessary for our full maturation into adulthood. It's required for having mature relationships, especially those that include sex. We get to become the empathic, compassionate, and understanding parents we always desired to have as children towards the child inside of us. By honoring our inner child, we get to restore in us the innocence with which we saw, felt, and experienced the world as children, prior to any of our childhood pain. We get to reap the benefit of emotionally mature and satisfying relationships, full of both intimacy and play.

We become more childlike in the sense that we see ourselves and each other through the eyes of our innocence, and children don't care about things like race, creed, color, status, sex, or orientation. They don't care about looks. They don't objectify each other. They only care about the person underneath those things. When connected with our innocence, anytime our conditioned mind starts to sexually objectify another, we'll remember that there's also a child inside of them, a child no different than the one inside us. We'll see their innocence, rather than just their body, and we'll remember that every person was once a child and every child deserves love. We have the power to be that kind of loving force in the world, towards ourselves and each other. It's reborn in us through our work with our inner child, through this restoration of our inner innocence.

One of my favorite ways of staying connected with my inner child is by using an old printed photo of myself from when I was about four or five years old. My favorite photo to use is the picture my mother took of me on my first day of school. White collar short-sleeve shirt, navy blue shorts, light-up power ranger shoes, I was ready to take on the world. Just looking at it starts to reconnect me with him; how he felt when I was him, what he loved, what was important to him, how he feels now.

I keep this photo with me throughout my day, looking at it periodically just to make sure that I'm checking in with him consistently. Sometimes I'll even close my eyes and connect with him visually. Most of the time he looks just like the little boy in the photo, but sometimes he looks a little different. I'll observe him, see what he's up to, explore his world and maybe even inspire a conversation with him. "Hey buddy, how are you feeling today? How's your heart?" Or, "what are you up to there?" Anything just to get him talking. He tells me all kinds of things, as children tend to do when they feel safe. You know how kids are when they get to sharing, they don't hold anything back.

Other times when I check in on him, I'll find him hiding in a closet or playing by himself. Sometimes he won't respond to my attempts to connect with him and that's how I know he's needing more of my presence and tenderness. Sometimes he wants to be held, sometimes he wants to be listened to and reassured, and sometimes he just wants me to be there spending time with him. It's always different but having this photo with me and checking in with him throughout the day allows me to have a pulse on how he's feeling in any given moment.

It also allows me to connect with him preemptively, especially if I know I'm stepping into a very "adult situation" like a big meeting, a serious conversation, a coaching call, or even love-making. Having this connection with him allows me to properly prepare him for any life situation that he may not fully understand and therefore react to from fear (as adults, we experience this as anxiety), just like I would make the time to properly prepare my son for things like plane rides, vacations, meeting new people, and stepping out into public. Having this photo with me (in my pocket, in my wallet, in the pages of a book I'm reading, etc.) makes it so much easier for me to see my inner child as soon as it's there for me to go inward and connect with him.

Another favorite practice of mine that I feel is essential for connecting with my inner child is what I like to refer to as mirror therapy. Mirror therapy isn't limited to our inner child by any means. It can be utilized to connect with every aspect of ourselves, but it's especially useful here. What I like to do is stand in front of the bathroom mirror, look myself directly in the eyes and picture my inner child looking back at me. As I eye gaze with him, I simply allow myself to feel whatever is there for me to feel; love, sadness, joy, delight, hurt. Most importantly, what this does is really get me in the presence of my own innocence.

Often, I find myself in front of the mirror when my inner child is afraid that he did something wrong, or that he did something unintentionally that hurt someone he loves. In the mirror I am able to reassure him that he didn't do anything wrong and explain to him what actually happened. I remind him that he's safe and that no matter what unfolds in our external world, I've got his back and will one hundred percent always be there looking after him. Other times I find him with a big, adorable smile on his face. In those moments, I simply receive his heart, his joy, and his innocent love for people, and it fills my heart. In those moments I tell him how proud of him I am, how much fun it is playing with him each and every day, and how much I delight in our time together. He loves hearing those things. It seems to only accentuate his already joyful demeanor.

Mirror therapy is epic for truly being in the presence of our inner child. It's so simple too. It opens our hearts to fully see and receive ourselves for who we are on the most basic and fundamental level. What could be more potent medicine than that? Don't be afraid to write to your inner child either. You may not have been fully literate by the time you were four or five, but you will certainly receive the energetics of it. Start out with something like, "Dear little one...," and then just let it rip. Go ahead and lavish love on your innocence. You know it's working when it brings tears to your eyes.

Last thing I want to say here is that part of our role as men is to protect the innocence. While that certainly means the children of our world, it also means the child within us. Building a relationship with our inner child allows us to more easily see and understand the child in ourselves and others. Given that everyone in our ever-growing world has an inner child, that's pretty much invaluable. When we become developed in reparenting our own inner child, we'll be available to recognize when the people in our lives are expressing on behalf of their inner child. That means we'll be available to show up compassionately for their innocence. This is a tremendous power to have in a world full of people that have no idea they even have an inner child. To be with another in the middle of their emotional experience and soothe them with compassion is truly a superpower. This isn't about rescuing or pretending like you're Mother Teresa. It's about having compassion for the fact that inside we are all children and all deserving of love.

We can offer ourselves and each other tremendous opportunities to heal through this inner child work and therefore embody more of our innocence, which is only going to make our world a more delightful and fun place to live. Be the type of parent to your inner child that you would want your children to have. When I first started this work, any time my inner child would feel hurt by something I would find myself saying things like, "god, this is so stupid" or "ah, I hate this. Don't be such a baby." Until one day it dawned on me that I would *never* talk to a real child like that. I would never belittle their emotions or make them feel less than. So why was I doing that to my inner child? Something to consider as you journey forth in this area.

Restoring our inner innocence will undoubtedly impact our world for the better. Seeing each other through the eyes of our innocence will only ever invite more love, compassion, kindness, and grace into our adult relationships. It will allow us to assume our role as protectors of innocence, as well as allow us to show up as men in our relationships, especially in the bedroom. You have no idea of the true power and potency of this work, so, it kind of goes without saying that I am inviting you to step into it wholeheartedly. Don't worry about other people finding out that you have a relationship with your inner child. I promise it will only make you a better lover, a more empathic husband, a more compassionate father, and a more loving man. Your wife and children will be better off because of it. Be brave, but especially savor the delight of allowing your inner child to shine. Because that's the you before any of your conditioning. That's the you that will awaken humanity to remember the innocence with which we are all born.

When we're in tune with our inner child, we're inherently available to see the innocence of others. That means every time our mind goes to sexually objectify another, whether in person or online, we'll remember that we're actually sexually objectifying an innocent child. We'll remember the innocence that dwells not only within us but within every human being that we encounter, no matter their age or background. Our interactions with the opposite sex will stem less from our unresolved childhood pain and more from our genuine desire to love, serve, and honor the feminine. We'll relate to our partners as empowered women, while also holding space for their inner innocence. Heal the boy and the man arises, the one that's capable of honoring sex and our underlying sexuality as sacred. Bring forth the part of your innocence that loves everybody, as all children do. Being connected to this innocence makes it that much easier for the most creative force in the universe go to work for love instead of fear.

Chapter 9

Tools for Reconnecting with Our Sexual Innocence

Just as our innocence was present for our first day of school, the first time we fell in love, our first kiss, and many other of our "first" young life experiences, our innocence was also present the first time we discovered our sexuality. Typically, what leads us to explore ourselves sexually is a healthy mix of genetic programming and innocent curiosity. Our bodies become endowed with a creative energy previously unknown to us and we instinctually begin investigating. The innocence with which we discover our sex energy is no different than the innocence with which we discover anything.

As crazy as it might sound, the same inner child that I spoke about in the previous chapter was absolutely present for our first sexual experience, whether that experience was one that we shared with someone else or one that we shared only with ourselves. Our sexuality is inherently innocent in nature, just as we are, but so many of us have lost our ability to see it this way. Embarking on this journey of rediscovering our sexual innocence, its natural existence prior to our early introduction to shame, is essential to our awakening. There are a few key practices that will help us tremendously in accomplishing our mission. Yes, they will require a little bit of bravery and a willingness to get a little uncomfortable, but as we all know, a little bit of bravery can go a very long way.

If it's not obvious by now with how many times I've mentioned it in this book, breath is an invaluable tool for not only reconnecting with the truth of our sexual innocence but also reconnecting with our higher-self. Deep, full, intentional belly breathing is the primary key to a relaxed nervous system, and it's only through a relaxed nervous system that we're capable of communing with our higher-self (or whatever you want to call it) experientially. It's what brings us out of our mind and into our body where we can tap into the greater wisdom of our heart.

Breathwork has a direct and immediate impact on our vibration. It's a tool with which we can consciously raise our vibration in any moment; whether that's at home in meditation, out in the world during our day to day life, at work, in the middle of bringing to life an inspired creation, or while making love. Our breath is an incredibly underutilized tool. The practice of breathing seems too simple to warrant its efficacy. How could something that's free, readily available around the clock, inherent to our humanity, and sitting right underneath our nose make such a dramatic impact on the quality of our lives? It's quite the conundrum, but it's especially significant to this conversation around sex, sex energy, and sexual desire.

I do intentional, intuitive breathwork nearly every single day, many times multiple times a day. It raises my in-the-moment vibration to that of my higher-self while simultaneously grounding me in my body. I utilize it especially when tapping into my creativity, like the kind of creativity it took to write this book. Every day before I sit down to write I breathe, relax my nervous system, allow my vibration to naturally rise. I prepare my vessel (my body) to receive the energy of my higher-self. I practice the same intentional breathing in the bedroom while making love with my beloved. Being connected to our breath and body during the act of love-making is essential to accessing the transcendental power of sex. If we're not fully present in our body, the magic simply isn't going to happen.

You would think experiencing something so regularly would make the experience itself less potent, like needing more caffeine to experience the same buzz, but it doesn't. The pleasure that's available for us to open-heartedly receive through our love-making is beyond anything you could ever imagine. Pleasure, if we allow it to be, can be just as much a profound spiritual teacher as pain. Unlike pain, pleasure is difficult for us to receive. That may seem counterintuitive, but it's true. We have been conditioned to believe that feeling pleasure is somehow a bad thing, and that anyone who shamelessly allows themselves to receive pleasure could only be a pervert. Before I reconnected with my sexual innocence, pleasure was something I was ashamed of, something I never wanted to be seen enjoying, something that made me incredibly uncomfortable. Desiring pleasure or even entertaining it from a place of curiosity left me feeling incredibly embarrassed and ashamed. I judged myself any time the desire to feel pleasure crossed my mind. Thank you, Catholicism! But pleasure is healing, and pleasure in unison with our breath is an undeniable vehicle for life-changing transformation.

As much as we're meant to channel our sex energy towards heart-centered creations that then go on to better our world, we're also meant to receive our sex energy for what it truly is; a sacred, spectacular, and powerful energy designed to deliver us pleasure. Equal parts my friends; equal parts pain and pleasure. The only issue being that we've become more comfortable with pain than we have pleasure. Pain is familiar, something everyone feels, often a point of relatability. We're all familiar with the conversation, the one where two people take turns sharing their life problems. We can relate to each other's pain, and when we do, it makes us feel connected to one another. Our bodies are much more comfortable with pain because they're used to feeling it; it's known, certain, a sure thing. The rest of the world seems to agree with this as well. How many times have you heard someone tell you, "life is hard," as in, get over it and accept that life is mostly full of struggle with a few blips of happiness in between?

We're so ashamed of feeling pleasure that when we do

intentionally seek it out, which is natural for us to do, we end up experiencing it through mostly distorted means, void of any real sense of connection or love. Pornography is a great example of this, but so is hooking up with other people under the influence of alcohol. We desperately want to experience pleasure, yet we have to numb ourselves to receive it. We feel such shame around receiving pleasure that we often attempt to hide it, causing us to delve into the shadows of our sexuality as opposed to owning pleasure as an aspect of our birthright. We don't need to feel such shame around receiving the pleasure that our bodies were designed to feel. All we really need to do is breathe. Breath is our simplest and most powerful means of receiving the innocent pleasure of our sex energy, and we certainly don't need to be having sex in order to feel it.

It just so happens that sex is the perfect analogy for life. How you do sex is how you do anything. How do you do sex? When it comes to sex are you:

- Present? (all of your awareness here in this present moment, fully in your body, not thinking about anyone or anything else, making eye contact, really seeing your partner, present to every touch, every sensation, every emotion)
- Listening? (connected to your intuition, listening for intuitive guidance, aware of your partner's desires/needs)
- Open-hearted? (allowing your sex energy to move through every part of your body, not just your sex organs, connected emotionally, passionate, fully involved, in the presence of your beloved's love for you and your love for her)
- Taking your time? (approaching the act with zero rush and zero attachment to an end goal, pausing from time to time, allowing the space to unfold naturally)
- Relaxed? (breathing deeply, allowing your body to move

in ways that it's inspired to, continuously relaxing the tension in your body, aware of what your body is feeling)

- Setting sacred space? (burning sage, lighting candles, diffusing essential oils, preparing your sanctuary for this sacred act, cleaning up the clutter, etc.) More on this in Chapter 15!
- Setting your intentions? (how you desire to feel, what you desire to create, what this co-creation of love is being directed towards, what purpose it's meant to serve, what you desire to transform, what you desire to heal and/or celebrate)
- Courting the divine? (inviting in your higher-self, your guides, angels, and spirit helpers)

When we reconnect with our breath and relax into our physical body, we become fully present with the experience of our body and merge with the blissful sensations of our sex energy. We also allow ourselves to be present to and hold space for our beloved's experience. When we continue to consciously breathe and relax further, we surrender into our sex energy all together, allowing it to relocate us to an experiential reality beyond our 3D space and time. We transcend our physicality and merge with the energy of our source, the euphoric oneness that pervades every living thing throughout the entire universe. Hence why we can get so lost in this space, so engulfed by it. Time itself seems to stand still.

By introducing breath into this sacred space, we naturally come to receive the true energy of our Source, or what I call God. Mostly thanks to religious dogma, we've all but abandoned the notion of God being something inside of us, but that is exactly what I am sharing with you here. Sacred sex is a real-life spiritual means for experiencing God within, through the vehicle of our body. All we have to do is breathe, set our intention, relax, and surrender into it.

How we do sex is how we do life. If we're tense, anxious, barely breathing and in our head, we're more than likely not going to surrender into receiving pleasure, and we're certainly not going to experience God. The same is true for life. For instance, if we're creating on our laptop while we're tense, anxious, barely breathing and stuck in our logical minds, then we're more than likely not going to receive the true pleasure that comes with creativity. And yes, you guessed it, we're certainly not going to experience God in the creative process.

Breathwork is one of the most influential and valuable tools I have ever discovered for fully relaxing the body into receiving pleasure. It works for both our creative process as well as our love-making. It's a powerful way to connect in and merge with our sex energy, and therefore, receive the pleasure of it. If you haven't already taken the hint, get yourself enrolled in some kind of breathwork class or start practicing intuitively. I don't have the space to walk you through breathwork exercises in this book, nor am I the most qualified person to do so. Recently I read a great book by Dan Brulé called *Just Breathe*. It's the perfect starting point for anyone interested in learning more about breathwork. It also contains many different techniques and practices.

The good news is, breathwork is more mainstream today than it's ever been. Take advantage of this. Go above and beyond to expand yourself in this area. Most of the practices are quite simple yet yield profound benefits. You'll find for yourself that the more you practice the more you'll have conscious control of your breathing and therefore your nervous system, vibration, and sex energy. I just let you in on one of the simplest yet most profound keys to the spiritual kingdom. Take me up on it.

Beyond breathwork is a practice that I personally love for anyone desiring to reconnect with their sex energy from a place of innocence. It's called a lingam massage and it's pretty much exactly as it sounds. It's a massage for your lingam (a spiritual term for your penis). Unlike masturbating where we typically attach our pleasure to sexual imagery, whether in our mind or on a screen, quickly build tension and then physically release, a lingam massage teaches us to relax, detach from our mind, and detach from the end goal of ejaculation. It's an intentional space for us to practice breathing and relaxing into pleasure. It's also a powerful tool for reconnecting with our sex energy, for those of you that are still confused as to what that is.

The goal is to relax, breathe, and receive pleasure while continuously letting go of the tension in your body. It's a super simple practice that you can try from the comfort of your own home. It goes like this, set some sacred space for yourself where you can have privacy and silence. Put on some noise canceling headphones if you have them. Bring the same level of intention to this space as you would love-making with your beloved. Burn some sage, set your intentions, invite in your higher-self, and go from there. Then use a topical oil of your choice and apply it to your lingam. Massage yourself until you become erect. On a sliding pleasure scale where zero is completely flaccid and ten is ejaculating, you want to keep yourself at a consistent seven or eight.

As you massage yourself just notice your tendencies around receiving pleasure. Do you clamp down with tension or are you able to stay relaxed and open? Is your breathing relaxed and deep or shallow and strained? Are you unconsciously holding your breath? Is your mind fixated on sexual imagery or are you free to contemplate whatever you desire? Are you allowing your sex energy to move through your entire body or are you keeping it limited to your genitals? When it gets to an eight or nine do you feel that you need to release or can you pause, breathe, relax and keep going? How much pleasure are you willing to receive? Where is your cap before you have to throw in the towel and release? Do you have to release in order to feel complete? Or can you refrain from ejaculating and still feel just as satisfied?

Notice everything. Observe yourself and your programmed relationship to your sex energy. Most importantly, feel your sex energy. Take this time to get so related to this energy that you'll never again mistake it for anything else. Get to know it, play with it, send it to specific points in your body, concentrate it in your third eye. Remember to breathe. Breathe this energy from your lingam up into your heart. When you're ready, surrender into your sex energy entirely and allow it to bathe you in its rapture. Allow your sacred life force to deliver you into the hands of God, which are of course, already inside you.

Practice as often as you're guided to but don't be surprised if you're blown away by your first session. My recommendation is to not ejaculate, at least not for the first few sessions, until you can relate to ejaculation as an optional experience as opposed to something that needs to happen in order for you to feel fully satisfied. Remember to connect all of this with your breathing. Deep, full, relaxed belly breathing. There's no time limit here, so don't rush. Give yourself the time you need to allow the magic to happen. On average, it only takes a man about two minutes to reach ejaculation. Give yourself at least fifteen minutes, thirty is even better, before deciding whether or not to keep going or complete the exercise.

This practice will not only make you a great lover, but it will also allow you to access and heal your sexual trauma and shame. It will allow you to restore the innocence with which your sexuality was founded and free you up to channel your sex energy through the sacred space of your heart. Don't be surprised if you feel emotional. Once your heart cracks open, anything is possible. You may tap into some emotional pain or broken heartedness from the past that's desiring to be acknowledged, felt, and released. Or, you may find yourself in such a state of awe and gratitude that you burst into tears. Both scenarios are appropriate. Once you set sacred space, anything goes. Just breathe, relax, and keep yourself at a consistent seven or eight and let the rest take care of itself. I find for myself that I end up going into a space of prayer, a meditative state where I'm sending my sex energy as a blessing to loved ones, the earth, and those people that I know are suffering the most.

It goes without saying that you can practice this exercise with your beloved. It requires presence and communication, the rules being that the two of you must maintain eye contact throughout the entire experience. Because it's no longer your hand coordinating the exercise, you will have to communicate with her what feels good and what doesn't, along with your number on the sliding pleasure scale. For instance, if you get to a nine and you're about to release, you'll have to let her know and request a moment to pause. If her massaging is too intense, you'll have to request that she slow down, relax her grip, or apply more oil.

It's a wonderful practice in intimacy and requesting what we need, as I am certain the two of you will discover for yourselves. Work with each other rather than against each other. Communicate clearly and graciously, with love. Remember, keep eye contact at all times. Allow your two separate perspectives to merge into one unified awareness. After you've practiced together a few times, try communicating without words. Communicate with your eyes, with your energy. Go beyond words.

If you can learn to relax and breathe in the sex space, you'll be able to relax and breathe in any space. This isn't just about sex, creating, or learning how to receive pleasure. It's a metaphor for life. This practice and the gifts that come from it will contribute to every area of your life. You will develop a heightened awareness of your sex energy and learn to interact with it and direct it in a way that's beneficial to you and others. As a biproduct of your creations (both in and outside of the bedroom), your positive impact on the world will become even more potent and powerful. Ultimately you will learn how to direct your sex energy in service to love while embodying the highest expression of your sexual nature.

Practice. It's an ever-ongoing refinement but you can progress by leaps and bounds with these two practices alone; breathwork and lingam massage. They are not all the keys to the kingdom but believe me when I tell you that they are one hell of a start. My encouragement here is don't believe me. Explore these practices for yourself and come to your own conclusions. Things like breathing and massaging ourselves are often so simple and so close to home that we easily overlook them. Yet sometimes our most powerful resources for expansion are right in front of us, we've just allowed ourselves to believe that it couldn't possibly be that simple. Let it be that simple, but don't take it for granted. Commit to a practice and stick with it.

Chapter 10

Hungry for Intimacy

I watched a video last week about a man struggling with ED, erectile dysfunction. His story went a little something like this. For the purposes of this share, I'll call this man Steve. Steve had been in a committed and faithful marriage for seventeen years, twelve of which were sexless. Yes, that's right, twelve years without sex. Most of us can't even imagine going twelve days without sex, let alone twelve years. One day something dawned on Steve. He finally woke up to the realization that he felt like he was slowly dying inside, and that if he didn't do something dramatic about it immediately, he was likely going to die, at least on the inside where it really matters. So, he divorced his wife, a long time coming from his perspective, and embarked on a new, exciting, and grand adventure of being a fifty-something-year-old bachelor. The world was his oyster and after twelve years of abstinence, let's just say Steve was single and ready to mingle. The only hiccup was, in the midst of tying up loose ends with the divorce, Steve was diagnosed with prostate cancer.

Okay, certainly not the worst kind of cancer a man can have, and definitely one with a good prognosis, especially when caught at an early age. The surgical procedure that Steve had to remove the cancer from his prostate rendered him impotent. If you don't know what that means, it simply implies that no matter what Steve did to "get it up," he couldn't achieve an erection. Based on the doctor's diagnosis, it was possible that Steve may never achieve an erection again. As you can imagine, Steve was devastated. Not only was he not going to be exploring the boundaries of his newfound sexual freedom, but he might never be capable of having sex again.

As destiny would have it, Steve met a woman a short time

later. They went on a few dates here and there until things started getting serious. Steve knew he had to come clean about his condition, but he was terrified by the thought of being rejected for it, let alone the idea of having his manhood laughed at. Despite his many fears, Steve went for it anyway, certain it would be the end of what had already been a deeply satisfying relationship.

Turns out the woman Steve was dating was shockingly understanding and open to exploring intimacy with him despite his condition. Steve was really hoping for a miracle here and had already attempted nearly every trick in the book to make "it" happen. His attempts came to a screeching halt the moment he sucked his left testicle up into a penis pump trying to get hard. The pain and embarrassment of the moment broke his heart open. Steve surrendered into the inevitable. He sobbed in his beloved's arms while she held him closely. What Steve described next is my reason for sharing this story with you. After surrendering into the fact that it was never going to happen, they both laid back into the bed together and began talking. Talking led to kissing, kissing led to touching, and touching led Steve like a runaway train into a deeply fulfilling experience of intimacy, unlike anything he had ever experienced before.

Now, I know what you're thinking. No, the intimacy Steve and his beloved shared did not miraculously fill Steve's penis with blood. Instead, these two lovers spent hours exploring intimacy, ecstasy, connection, pleasure, and sensuality without penetration. Erection taken off the table, and therefore ejaculation, there was nothing to rush off to. Because of this, Steve was granted the deepest experience of intimacy he had ever experienced in his entire life, bringing tears to his eyes as he shared about it on stage.

Later, he went on to share that the seemingly unfortunate circumstances that led to his ED were actually the greatest blessing he had ever received. Steve was finally able to satisfy a deep, inner yearning for intimate connection that he hadn't had access to before. He, like most men, thought he just wanted to have really great sex. When really, Steve, like every man, just wanted to feel the deep, inner satisfaction that comes from experiencing real intimacy. Steve was desiring to share the deepest aspects of himself with another, and the pleasure he received from doing so, was far better than anything a simple erection could offer him.

We are all like Steve in our own way. We think sex is what we desire, when in reality, intimacy is what we're really after. Intimacy is what fills our cup, more so than even our most outlandish sexual experiences. Sure, it comes with a natural maturity, but it's ultimately where we land. We're hungry for connection, we're hungry for a closeness that only real intimacy can provide. Most men go their entire lives without experiencing this intimacy. We learn to place value on other things like developing our career or making a lot of money, because we haven't ever felt the deep inner satisfaction that comes with genuine intimacy.

Intimacy is scary. It's not so put together. It's certainly not as safe as clocking in and clocking out just to earn a paycheck. It's the realest of the real, our deepest inner truths, the things we're scared to share because of how it might be interpreted or what others might think. Intimacy is a fundamental desire for every human being on Earth, not only men. We all want to feel deeply connected and known for who we are underneath the mask. We all long to be seen, yet it's the thing that frightens us the most.

Intimacy is almost like this mythological word that gets thrown around conceptually without any concrete evidence to back its existence. That's because, what's more important than the way we choose to define intimacy, existing as a mostly logical concept in the mind, is the way that we experience intimacy with our body. Like it or not, most of us did not receive the nurturing we needed in our young lives to feel fully safe in our physical body. For that reason, genuine intimacy for most men feels like something along the lines of attempted double homicide. In other words, it feels like death to the ego, death to our personality, and most importantly, death to the mask we put on every single day before stepping out into the world. Who are we really beneath this mask? Why should that man be exiled from love-making if he is who we really are?

Maybe a better question to lead with is "What does intimacy feel like to me?" A question that in and of itself implies being connected to our physical body and the emotions inside of it. Intimacy with another is not even a possible until we're first connected with our own inner world. Sure, we can listen, but listening alone doesn't leave us in the presence of intimacy. To create real intimacy is to share ourselves openly and honestly. To share ourselves openly and honestly, we need only look into our inner world, at what's happening within our physical body.

Close your eyes. Take a deep breath and look right now into your own inner world. Yes, right now. I'll wait. What are you feeling? Curiosity? Boredom? Excitement? Joy? Sadness? Peace? This is where intimacy really begins, by looking inward and connecting with what's happening in our body. That's it. That's all it really is. An in the moment check in with our physical body and an honest and open revealing of what's there. Kind of simplifies this whole intimacy thing, doesn't it?

Early on, when I was first trying to share my inner world with others, I found it helpful to start by sharing my physical sensations. My beloved would ask me something like, "what's on your heart?" I would pause, close my eyes, scan my body with my awareness, and describe what it was I was feeling physically. I would say something like, my chest feels tight, or my brain feels a bit cloudy, or my stomach feels a little queasy.

Then together we would go the next layer deeper. "Do you know why you're feeling what you're feeling?" I feel tightness in my chest because I'm a little hurt that we haven't had any time together today. My brain feels a bit cloudy because I've been so wrapped up in work and tied to technology all day. My stomach feels queasy because I'm a little nervous for this meeting I'm leading tomorrow. It's kind of a big deal. Then, the next layer deeper. Tell me about your hurt. What was it that you were so intentionally working on today? Have you talked with your inner child about the meeting? And so on.

To express honestly and openly and therefore begin the process of creating intimacy, we need only be connected to our physical body. If we're not first connected to the inner workings of our own physical body, how can we ever expect to engage intimately with the body of another, especially through something as sacred as love-making? We simply cannot, not really anyway. How do we connect intimately with our body? Great question! For me, I connect intimately with my body through both stillness and movement. When I'm in stillness, eyes closed, breathing intentionally, it's quite easy for me to connect with what I'm feeling inside. I may not yet understand why I'm feeling the way I am, but I can at least pinpoint the emotion and start from there.

I have a similar experience when I'm exercising, stretching, or simply doing breathwork. All of these movements grant me access to my emotions and where in my body I am feeling that emotion. For the most part, on any given day, men do everything but be with themselves in this way. Usually our schedules are so packed that we're moving from one action item to the next not really knowing our ass from a hole in the ground. I don't actually know what that means but I've heard it expressed many times throughout my life. I take it to mean that we don't actually know what's going on in our inner world because we haven't yet paused long enough to explore it.

And rightfully so. Our external world demands our attention constantly. The few times in our week when it's not in demand, we quickly find ways to distract ourselves from looking inward; food, video games, movies, television, social media, socializing, cat videos on YouTube. Not distracting ourselves and making time to go inward is what allows us to offer our inner world outward, the result being intimacy. It seems simple enough, but the cold reality is that most people alive on our planet right now are disconnected from what's happening emotionally inside of them, especially men. Now that we know that, all there is to do is go inward and see what's there. After we discover what's happening in our inner world, it's only about embodying a little bit of bravery in sharing what we find.

Sometimes the most honest answer to an inquiry about what's happening in our inner world is, "I don't know." That answer is perfect when it's honest. When our answer is genuinely, I don't know, the invitation becomes to pause, close our eyes, and look right now. I find I'm most hesitant to share my inner world when I'm feeling disconnected from it myself. Put on the spot, I sometimes put pressure on myself to "get it right" rather than take a moment of silence to go inward and investigate. Because I want to connect, I'll look for something, anything, even if I'm not completely convinced it's true. The continuation of questioning from my beloved can easily have me feel confused and frustrated.

If I'm honest, I'm never actually frustrated with her. I'm frustrated with myself that I'm either unaware of what's going on emotionally inside of me or didn't ask for what I needed, which was just a few moments of silence to go inward before answering. Sometimes I can do it right there, look within and express what I'm feeling in my body. Other times it's authentic for me to ask for a moment to scan my body. I certainly encourage you to explore all of your different options.

Often, our woman can pick up on the presence of an emotion

in our physical body well before we can. While we're fumbling around in our heads, they're the one to point out something fishy going on in our inner world. I used to hate it when this would happen. I would react with something like, "Oh, so now you think you know my emotions better than me?" I felt threatened by the fact that it was actually true. Now I see it as an invitation to pause and drop in with my body. This is one of those things that still has me feeling a bit uncomfortable to this day, but I've learned that surrender is the key. When I fight it, it's only because I don't want to give in to the fact that she's right and reveal myself vulnerably.

In short, sex is not really what you're after here. Connection is. When you explore your inner world to the point where you're able to access your emotions and share them openly, you won't ever have to worry about sex. Sex will be the cherry on top, because your heart will already be full from the intimacy present in your relationship. Full-hearted sex is what we're really after here. When our hearts are open from having experienced real intimacy, the love-making just flows naturally as it's meant to. Our bodies become free to connect with each other in the ecstatic ways that they're so brilliantly designed to. Sex becomes both an emotional and a spiritual experience. That's when it feels really juicy, and both of you are left in the aftermath of love-making completely blown away, contemplating how what you just experienced is even possible.

We're hungry for intimacy, not sex. We long to feel deeply connected to others, especially our lovers. We long to experience love in all its forms. We do that in love-making by entering into the ceremony with an open heart, with not a single aspect of ourselves tucked away or hidden. This is the new frontier of sex, passionate love-making where our hearts intertwine and dance their ecstatic dance. You don't need to look any further than your physical body and the emotions inside of it to dance this divine dance. Aren't you relieved it's that simple? Our ability to create intimacy with one another is only ever a reflection of our willingness to first experience intimacy with ourselves. That, my friends, is the nectar of a truly fulfilling life, let alone a wildly satisfying sex life.

Chapter 11

Restoring the Heart

Heartbreak is real. Depending on how we relate to it, it has the capacity to be a tremendous catalyst for intimacy or our justification for closing off our heart indefinitely. How open we are to processing our heartbreak (aka feeling it fully) ultimately determines how open we are to love, especially the kind of love we find in love-making. We've all had experiences of heartbreak, from being dumped by our first crush to letting go of a vision that we thought for sure was part of our purpose. Heartbreak is a natural part of being human. When we allow it to crack us open, it's sometimes the most beautiful part about being human. Humans are hardwired for emotion. No matter how hard we try, there's simply no escaping it. Our emotions come and go as they please, seemingly of their own accord, unconcerned for whether or not it's good timing. Our relationship to our emotions makes all the difference when it comes to living with an open heart.

This chapter is intentionally titled restoring the heart because it's the global mission of our time. This time is about bringing the heart back into the areas of our lives where we've stamped it out for the sake of profit, progress, personal gain, power, and selfish pleasure, especially in our sex life. To succeed at our mission, we must develop a healthy, working, and constructive relationship with our emotions. We must honor our emotions and celebrate them as an extraordinary part of what it means to be human, not something to fix, change, rush through, avoid, suppress, or condemn in any way.

We've become masters at condemning our emotional body. Trained early on to invalidate our emotions, we judge them for making us feel weak. We judge ourselves for having emotions in the first place. As adults, emotions make us squirmy. They make us feel like we're not in control of our life or body. We go to workshops, attend courses, and hire coaches to strengthen our mind, anything to give us a leg up on our emotions. Why has suppression become our primary means for relating to our emotional body?

We all know the traditional masculine archetype of the stoic, silent, lone wolf of a man. The one that's totally self-sufficient, a-emotional, and doesn't need a damn thing from you, me, or anyone else in order to survive. Those tough, durable, weathered, rugged sons of bitches that we've worshipped everywhere from our family dynamics to bigtime professional athletes to our beloved Hollywood screen actors like Clint Eastwood, Sylvester Stallone, Arnold Schwarzenegger, Liam Neeson, Samuel L. Jackson, Vin Diesel, Tom Hardy, and Jason Statham. We've generally accepted this archetype as our modern-day blueprint for masculinity; muscles, money, and mojo. The most important piece of all being, never show your emotions, unless of course those emotions are anger and aggression.

While we certainly do feel anger, aggression, and even rage at times, there's so much more to a man's heart than these elementary expressions. Even those men that are charismatic, talkative, and have lots of friends have more to their heart than they reveal. As men, we're comfortable talking about work, sports, politics, and women, but we're not at all comfortable revealing our emotions. We've conformed to a gender norm that's inauthentic to who we are, and we're all just waiting around for someone to give us permission to express ourselves vulnerably.

The masculine heart is pure in its essence. It's a divine protector, space holder, lover, and fierce warrior for truth. Every one of us is a king, warrior, priest, magician, and lover, but without the full activation of our heart, what difference does it make? A king without his heart is nothing more than a tyrant. A warrior without his heart, a killer. A priest without his heart, a fraud, the embodiment of false devotion. We've all heard the phrase, boys who don't cry shoot bullets. Maybe that's why men account for about 96% of all homicide perpetrators and 80% of all homicide victims worldwide. Hasn't our world seen enough of this kind of emotional expression?

The way that we teach our boys to relate to their emotions is directly related to the violence we're experiencing on a global scale. It's not always directed towards other people either. Three-fourths of the 800,000 people that take their lives every year are men. "Stop crying. Man up. Don't be such a pussy. That's gay." Expressions that impacted every one of us as a child, still hindering our ability to express our hearts vulnerably. Most men would rather die than let others know they're hurting. Many men already have. This is especially true when it comes to sharing our heartbreak.

Every single one of us has experienced heartbreak in our lifetime, but how many of us have actually given ourselves permission to feel it? How many of us have let our hearts be shattered into a million pieces? Most have not, because our conditioning says don't cry, be a man, and get over it. Most of us took the heartbreak we experienced and stuffed it down so deep that we hardly even notice it's there anymore. It lingers silently, constantly hindering our ability to give and receive love.

Emotional suppression isn't a selective process. When we suppress our heartbreak, we also suppress our joy, happiness, excitement, delight, cheerfulness, and enthusiasm. Suppressing one emotion suppresses them all. We cling to a middle ground, never too emotionally high and never too emotionally low. We flatline our emotional body and wonder why we have to go to such extremes to feel anything at all. When something happens that breaks our heart and we don't allow ourselves to feel it, that hurt gets trapped inside us.

Like a city under siege, we draw up our bridges, lock the gates, and arm the cannons. We think we're protecting ourselves from further pain but really, we've just trapped ourselves inside with it. We get so good at building walls and blocking people out that we end up living in relative isolation. We could be standing in a room full of people, even our closest friends and family, yet still feel utterly alone. Even though we're smiling, nodding, and getting along, the real us is trapped inside, our heartbreak still right there with us.

How is this related to sex? When we close our heart down in one area of life, we close our heart down to some degree or another in every area of life, including our sex life. Sex without emotion, without the complete presence of a fully open heart, is just two people rubbing parts hoping to generate enough friction for orgasm. Sure, it feels good. Orgasms are great, but the 10—20 seconds of heightened sensation is nothing in comparison to the timeless sensation of an orgasming heart. A sensation that requires no friction, no penetration, and no ejaculation whatsoever. When the heart orgasms from being overwhelmed by love, there's not even a desire for ejaculation. Instead of the energy being fixed in our genitals, it's allowed to move like blood through our bloodstream, igniting pleasure in every area of our body. We're left floating in the ecstasy of the eternal moment, no body, no mind, just love, pouring into us from every direction.

Yes, it sounds airy fairy, but when you experience it for yourself, you'll remember my words here. When your heart beckons you and you surrender to its rapture, you will never again settle for superficial sex. In fact, superficial sex will turn you off entirely. Because sex without a fully open heart, without the passionate fire of our emotions, is kind of like black coffee; stimulating but short-lived. Not only does it leave a bad taste in your mouth, but once the effects wear off, you feel worse than you did before.

Somewhere along the lines someone did something that broke your heart. The pain that you felt made you draw up your drawbridges, and you've been living in isolation ever since, fearful of that same heartbreak being inflicted upon you again. Close your eyes. Remember a time when you felt heartbroken. Take a few moments to conjure up the memory. Feel into where that energy is trapped inside your body. Go there. Access that part of your body with all of your presence and awareness. Invite the energy from where it is now into your heart. Coax it there with your focus.

When the energy hits your heart, surrender to it. Feel it, all of it. Allow the heartbreak to flow freely through you, holding nothing back. You've held onto this pain for long enough. Give yourself permission to let the heartbreak pass through you once more, this time without getting trapped or suppressed in any way. After the emotion passes, witness your heart naturally open again. Witness as it naturally expands to receive more love. You're stronger than you believe. Your heart was made to hold the heartbreak of the world inside of it. When we allow our heartbreak to reach into the most tender parts of us, something magical happens. It ignites our fire. Our pain turns to passion, and that passion drives us to be of service to the world.

When I first started my journey of restoring my heart, I had two spontaneous memories resurface to be reconciled and healed. The first was the first time I ever had my heart broken by a woman. It was young love, but real to me, nevertheless. I was obsessed with this girl, deeply infatuated with her from the moment I laid eyes on her. Call it chemistry, call it karma, call it whatever you want, when I looked at her my heart fluttered. I had courted her for nearly three years, from the time I was a freshman in high school to the time I was a junior. She was one class ahead and two years older.

We would flirt, spend hours on the telephone together, laugh, hold each other's gaze, but most importantly, we became close friends. She wore my jersey to the Friday night varsity football games and cheered me on from the bleachers.

One day out of nowhere, she asked me to the Sadie Hawkins Dance (the one where the girls ask the guys). I was shocked, flattered, intimidated, and excited all at once. This was it, the opportunity I had been waiting for, my chance to make it official with my high school sweetheart. The night of the big dance felt like a dream come true. It couldn't have been more perfect; pictures, dinner, party bus, the dance, all virtually flawless. The chemistry between us felt electric. As I made my way to the senior afterparty, I felt nervous. "Was this going to be the night?"

By the time I arrived, the energy of the evening had clearly shifted. The alcohol was in full effect. I tried my best to fit in, being the only junior amongst the senior crowd, but I didn't feel comfortable being there. If not for my date, I wouldn't have been there at all. Not long into the party, my date disappeared from my side. I played it cool trying to spot her, but I couldn't see her anywhere. After about an hour of entertaining meaningless conversations, I decided to go looking for her.

Slowing coming around the kitchen doorway, I was paralyzed by the sight of my high school sweetheart with another man's tongue half way down her throat. Worse yet, the tongue of a senior guy I hated. It was happening right there in front of me and about twenty other party goers. I could feel everyone's eyes slowly turn to me as they caught me entering the doorway. Shocked, devastated, confused, and embarrassed, I immediately turned, walked out of the kitchen and fell into the nearest sofa chair I could find. I didn't cry and I didn't react with anger. I just sat there in that sofa chair staring off into the distance feeling like my whole world had just been flipped upside down. "How could this have happened? How could I have been so naive?"

Nothing seemed to change after that experience. I left as early as I could the next morning and life just seemed to go on. I never once cried, nor did I share about it with any of my friends. When I saw her again at school the next week, I just ignored her and pretended I didn't care. But I did care, a whole lot for that matter. Inside I felt betrayed and embarrassed—not only was I heartbroken but now everybody in my school was gossiping about it. Not one tear, though. Not one stinking tear. My pride wouldn't let me. I made a powerful decision that day. I promised myself that I would never again open up my heart like that to a woman. It was too risky and too painful. My bridges came up, and my heartbreak traveled with me into every romantic relationship thereafter.

I was extremely clear with myself that the next time I got into a relationship, I would make sure it wasn't possible for me to get hurt like that again. The second memory that surfaced was from about a year later. A senior now, I decided to give love another try. Although tentative at first, I fell in love again, only this time even more so than before. At the time, I was going through a rough patch with my family. I had decided to break away from the Catholic church and branch out spiritually. I was interested in exploring myself and the emerging world of the New Age movement.

My family wasn't taking it so well, especially my mother. During those times, I leaned on my girlfriend and her family for comfort. They took me in when I felt cast out by my family. When my parents filed for bankruptcy in 2009, my girlfriend's parents supported me in transferring from a small division-three Christian college that I couldn't afford anymore, to a much larger division-one university. I felt a sense of acceptance from her family, one that I was longing for from my own, especially through those immensely challenging times.

Fast forward a few years and there we were planning the next stages of our lives together. I would go to Naturopathic medical school in Arizona and she would attend its sister college for the healing arts, conveniently just down the road. It seemed like the perfect plan, etched in stone. One weekend she went home to visit her family, something she did every so often. I didn't think anything of it. I went out that Friday night with some of our mutual friends and had a few drinks. I woke up the next morning to a phone call from my girlfriend. Dazed, confused, and still a little drunk from the night before, I answered the phone.

She opened the conversation by saying she had some bad news to share. The tone in her voice made it seem pretty serious. I immediately started running through the list of people that could have died. I never imagined it was our relationship that was dying. She went on to share that her feelings for me had shifted from romance to friendship, that she felt it was best for us to just be friends. Shocked, I begged her to reconsider, but she was clear. She had already spent the last twenty-four hours working out the details with her family. I hung up the phone having not only lost my best friend and what I believed to be my future wife, but also my surrogate family. To say that I felt heartbroken would be a dramatic understatement. More like shattered into a million pieces, not sure if I could ever pick them up. I did cry initially, probably because of the alcohol, but as soon as I got sober, my tears dried up.

The weeks and months that followed were pretty messy for me. She moved on much faster than I did and before I knew it, I was out at bars watching her flirt with other men. Occasionally she would get drunk and cry about how much she missed me. I would take care of her and make sure she got home safe, never letting things get physical. My heart was getting tossed around on spin cycle. I still loved her and of course wanted to be with her, so much so that I hung around far longer than I should have.

As much as I wanted to blame her for my pain, deep down I knew it was me that was holding onto it. By not feeling my heartbreak, I was able to stay in denial about the relationship being over. Twice now my heart had been broken by women I loved, and twice now I had refused to feel it. My romantic relationships that followed would suffer because of it. My repressed heartbreak was bubbling up to the surface as anger. I was mad at women. I dated for the convenience of sex and companionship, but my heart was nowhere near my sleeve. It was only after years of romantic union with my now beloved that I realized how much pain I was still holding onto.

My heart's revival came twelve long years after my initial heartbreak. Twelve years of suppressed emotion, broken relationships, bad romance, and unnecessary collateral damage. After twelve years, I was finally ready to honor my heartbreak and let it go. Sparked by some deep contemplation of my *Gene Keys*, the memories returned. Sitting in our kitchen in Southern California, I cried in my beloved arms, at times sobbing uncontrollably. My body shook and tremored as the pain surface. It was a somatic release like I'd never experienced before.

Twelve long years after my seeing my high school sweetheart kiss another man, I could finally see how closed off my heart had become to love. I felt like I was damaged goods, but as the pain passed, I felt myself becoming lighter. Gradually, I recovered the part of me that longed for romance. Trusting love again, I reopened my heart to let it all hit me. As my heart softened, our love-making deepened. That's when I first experienced a heart orgasm. Tears streamed down my face as I made love to my beloved. For the first time, I was receiving her, instead of protecting myself from her.

What past heartbreaks are you still holding onto? How are they impacting your life? Your relationships? Your sex life? If you give it some time, I bet you won't have to wait long until you can pinpoint those heartbreaking experiences. They're probably already there with you now. Holding on to heartbreak of the past is like drinking poison. It steals away any possibility of intimacy in the present. Until we feel it fully, our heartbreak travels with us everywhere we go, becoming a part of everything we do. We enter into sex either completely disconnected from our heart, using the act to fulfill a selfish desire, conceiving and creating more closed heartedness, or we enter into love-making guarded and tense, trying our best to protect our wounds.

Having experienced both superficial sex and heart orgasming love-making, it's not hard for me to recognize which one is more fulfilling. So much can happen in this sacred space of love-making. It's so much more than just friction, penetration, and ejaculation. It's two people merging and coming together as one, becoming the One. Sex is the most detailed and vast energetic exchange that you could possibly share with someone. When shared in a safe and trustworthy container, the act becomes a cataclysmic foreground for transformation.

We tend to resist the pain of our heartbreak at all costs. We strive instead for a superficial kind of pleasure. Like gerbils, we pedal the wheel round and round, chasing pleasure, running from pain, never getting anywhere. All the while robbing ourselves of the present moment. We think pain is bad and pleasure is good, pain something to run from and pleasure something to capture. We forget that pain is our ally, something that can continually crack open our heart. Within every heartbreak lies a gift, but it's only in being with our heartbreak that the gift is revealed; open heartedness, intimacy, connection, tenderness, love. It's through going back to the beginning and allowing ourselves to feel our initial heartbreak that we open the door to love. The pain is great, but the reward is a life lived from the sacred space of your heart. Your reward is feeling alive, like your heart getting revived by a defibrillator.

The last thing that I'll say here is that the body is always the last to heal. I spent years flowing in and out of personal and professional development courses, grasping aspects of my heartbreak with my mind. Rationally I understood what had happened, what I had made it mean, and how it was still impacting me in my day to day life. My rational understanding of the situation in no way helped me release the emotion still trapped in my body. My body was operating on its own time frame, and yours is too. Be gracious with it. Don't try to force your own healing. Everything occurs in its own time.

Our physical bodies are often the last part of us to go through their healing process because they're the densest of all of our bodies (mental, emotional, spiritual, etc.). What our bodies need in order to go through their healing process is simply safety. Give your body permission to go there by showing it that it's safe with you. It needs to know that if it starts to go into its healing process, you're not going to shut it down with substances or your mind. Go slow, take your time, don't rush your healing. Your awareness of the heartbreak is enough to signal to your body that you're ready to support it though its healing process.

If it helps, think of your body as something separate from you, the vehicle for your higher-self. Love it and give it what it needs to properly heal in its own way, in its own time. Listen to how it's asking to be nourished. This is an essential part of the work. So many lightworkers abandon their body because of how uncomfortable it can feel at times. Don't be one of those people. Stand up for your body to be fully healed regardless of how long it takes or how it looks in comparison to someone else's journey.

Chapter 12

Purposeful Sex

What's the purpose of sex? We know it feels good, that's pretty obvious, but from a spiritual perspective, what purpose does sex serve? From my personal exploration of this question, I've come to the conclusion that sex, and specifically the type of sex that I'm now calling love-making, serves four main purposes. The first is pretty self-explanatory: procreation. It's the process by which a man and a woman come together and create new human life, a child. Our physical body, initially forged by the sexual explosion of the masculine (sperm) and the receptive nature of the feminine (egg), becomes the vessel through which our spirit enters. From our parents, we inherit not only our DNA but also our early life perspectives, especially our perspective on sex. Our parents inherited this from their parents, their parents from their parents, so on and so forth. We're not eternally tied to our inheritance, however. Despite what modern science might tell you, biology is dynamic, DNA is dynamic. Just as our perspectives can change, our biology can too. Through the internal work we do as adults, we have the power to influence what we pass on to our children, both genetically and energetically, a power we ought to be utilizing consciously.

The type of sex we have matters. Our vibration during sex matters. Each time we engage in sex, something gets conceived, even when it's not a physical child. When it's not a physical child, we conceive energy. Think of this like energetic offspring. Energetic offspring are born from intention. This is still procreation, it's just not physical. When we merge with another in the sacred space of love-making, our energies get amplified one thousand-fold. They say that sound carries on for all eternity, continuing on as a vibration long after it can no longer be heard. Sex is no different. The ripple effect of our loving-making continues on long after the final act.

When two people making love direct their sex energy towards a single intention, that intention gets amplified. That's why it's often referred to as "sex magic." It's so powerful it seems like magic. Through our focused attention on a single intention, we can use this amplified energy field to bring our intentions to life. Our intentions can be as big or as small as we want them to be, just as long as they are genuine. We can intend things for ourselves, for our union, for our life, or our partner's life. The opportunity here is to utilize our love-making to conceive something meaningful, an intention that once manifested, will positively impact our lives.

We can also intend things beyond ourselves, beyond the two lovers sharing in this sacred act. What we conceive energetically can be strong enough to benefit all of humanity. Intentions of this size take on a form of their own. They become our prayers. We can pray for peace, for all people to know that they're worthy of love, for compassion and forgiveness, or for people to come home to their hearts and remember that they too are a beloved child of the universe. Again, what we intend on a large scale, what we pray for and conceive energetically, is completely up to us. Each prayer is unique, and each prayer impacts the collective in its own unique way.

I like to pray that each person alive on our planet discovers themselves worthy of grace. I pray that every man, woman, and child remember their inherent innocence, their divine birthright, the love from which they came, and their power to embody that love in life. Each time we make love with an intention of this size, our prayer gets cast out like a net wrapping itself around the Earth. It eventually makes its way all the way back to us. We too receive our own prayers. They are powerful. Prayers are healing. Our love-making can expand the impact of our prayers, allowing them to penetrate deeper into the collective heart of humanity.

The second purpose of love-making is for all of us to learn how to receive, in this case, receive pleasure. Our human psyche has been warped through generations of sexual repression to believe that we are either unworthy of receiving pleasure or that pleasure itself is somehow wrong or bad. Despite our conditioning, our bodies are hardwired for pleasure, just as they are emotion. Without our inherited conditioning around pleasure, all that remains is our body's God-given ability to receive it. Pleasure ought to be thought of as another part of a healthy human diet. It not only nourishes our body, but it also strengthens our spirit.

Some people construe us as more than a physical body. There's also our emotional body, mental body, and our energetic body. When we're making love and allowing ourselves to receive the pleasure of our love-making, we're actually supporting, nourishing, and strengthening our energetic body. Pleasure, especially orgasm, is energy, right? The energy of orgasm is incredibly powerful. When we bathe in that energy, and hold our focus on our energetic body, our energy body strengthens. Think of it like charging your phone. As brilliant as your phone is, without a charged battery, it's useless. Our bodies are similar, and love-making is one of the most powerful ways we can charge our battery. If our hearts aren't open to receive the pleasure, charging won't happen. We'll end up expending energy rather than charging up.

If we can learn to receive pleasure, in its purest and most potent form, then we can also learn to receive other things in life like support, guidance, prosperity, healing, clarity, and most of all, love. Love-making is a training ground for learning how to receive, but the application of what we learn applies everywhere in our lives. Let's say you have a really negative money story that you adopted from your parents. Your whole life you've believed that having money makes you a bad person, that to have money must mean that you took it from someone else.

Because of your story, you thought you had to choose between being a good person and having a lot of money. So, you, being who you are, chose to be a good person, but closed yourself off to receiving money. In the world we live in today, money is important. You need money to fulfill your life purpose. If you can't feed yourself and take care of your wellbeing, you're not going to thrive, and you're certainly not going to be in a position to serve powerfully. The whole pouring from an empty cup thing. Here's your opportunity to practice. Love-making is your playground for reopening your heart to prosperity. If you can learn to receive pleasure, then you can learn to receive money. Not only can you make prosperity your intention for love-making, but you can also allow the pleasure of the ceremony to amplify your heart's ability to receive it.

The more we allow ourselves to receive pleasure during love-making, the better we'll be at receiving pleasure from life. Remember, how you do sex is how you do anything. I'm talking about pausing that extra second to lean in and smell the roses, feeling that insect crawl up the back of your neck and instead of flicking it away, allowing its little legs to make your skin tingle. It's chewing a few moments longer to savor every flavor, listening to the birds serenade the morning air at sunrise, hugging a tree and feeling it hug you back, looking up at the stars at night in awe of the vast universe we're all a part of, looking in your lover's eyes and witnessing her magnificence. It's allowing ourselves to be fully hit by the beauty of life that's right here in front of us, all around us, living inside of us. It's receiving our own sacred essence, the being living inside this body, a divine creation of the cosmos. Receiving pleasure in this way often pushes us right up against our feelings of unworthiness. Leaning into the initial discomfort of receiving pleasure nudges us over the edge, so to speak, into the truth of how worthy and deserving we already are.

The third purpose of sex is healing. Sex is a profound space of healing when we allow it to be. The intensity of love co-created between two lovers can evoke from us anything that's not in alignment with love, things like our judgments towards ourselves, our guilt around past events, our fear of being fully seen and heard, or the pain of being betrayed by a close friend. All that can be brought to the surface during love-making. It's a true ceremony, and in ceremony, anything goes.

In life, shit happens. People get hurt. We feel hurt at times. We're never so spiritually evolved that we don't feel pain. We're all still human. In love-making we never know what might rise to the surface, but we do know that whatever does rise, we're going to love it. In fact, it rises during love-making because of our love. The presence of love is what has our body feel safe to release the pain. A container for such healing cannot be created through sex alone. It's takes a real commitment to someone, to all of someone, the good, the bad, and the ugly, and everything in between, to experience healing like this. Ultimately, the love that we co-create strips us raw before one another. Anything can be healed in the presence of that kind of love. Love-making is not only about our own personal healing. What we heal in ourselves, we heal within the world, something Marvin Gaye must have been onto when he fashioned the song *Sexual Healing*.

The fourth purpose of love-making is celebration. Love-making is our reward for choosing to open our hearts and live in a way that honors the sacred. It's one of the many perks of being alive, of being human. Aside from its distorted expressions, when we make love, we court the divine. We utilize our humanity to merge with something more, something bigger than our individuality. We celebrate being both human and divine, earthy and celestial, physical and ethereal. We're acknowledging that even though we're here living our very human lives, we're also a part of something bigger. We may not know what that "bigger" is, but we touch its essence during love-making. We remember what a privilege it is to be alive, to get to be here on this Earth, living this life. That life itself is a ceremony, sacred, and deserving of our celebration.

Life is short, here and gone in the blink of an eye, and while we're here, we tend to take it all far too seriously. Love-making is our space to loosen that up a bit. I am well aware of the suffering on our planet and the duality that comes with being human, but our suffering is only half of our story. The other half is our brilliance, our beauty, our majesty, and our tenderness. The human spirit is truly magnificent, and love-making is one way to celebrate this magnificence. Love-making is a tribute to love itself. It's paying homage to the love that created us, the love that lives inside us, the love that we all stem from. Our way of saying thank you to whomever we believe created us for this marvelous experience of being alive, we'll not let it go wasted. So, please, don't let it go wasted. Open your heart and celebrate the love you were made from. What better way could we possibly have to say thank you?

The purpose of sex is much bigger than you expected. It can be confronting at times to recognize and acknowledge this. We like to think of ourselves as small, insignificant people, irrelevant to the whole. When in reality, the opposite is actually true. The love that we are capable of creating and the impact that love can have on our world is beyond linguistic expression. When our hearts fully awaken this will become our primary purpose for love-making... conceiving love, gestating love, birthing love, nurturing love, raising love, and watching love take on a life of its own.

We have within us the power to create worlds, and how we choose to focus that power makes all the difference. The future awaits those that are ready to wield their creative powers in the name of love. Don't wait. Our future is only ever an imagined variation of now. Now is what we have, and now is the time we rise in love, and use our human superpowers to make love. Let this be the time when our collective love-making forever changes not only what it means to be a man, but also what it means to be a human. Let this be the gift we pass on to our children.

Chapter 13

Creating a Safe & Trustworthy Container

Every person regardless of race, color, creed, or sexual orientation has the right to enjoy sex as a natural expression of their humanity. We were born sexual beings and we will die sexual beings; it's a part of who we are. Negative social conditioning has long taught us to fear our sexuality. This fear has been passed down from one generation to the next since the dawn of recorded history. Fear evokes attraction, but it does nothing to open us to the ecstatic realms of sex. Instead, it closes down our hearts, preventing us from reaching them.

It beckons the question, who are we without this fear? What would happen if we let our walls down and started talking about sex openly? Would the world slip into a giant orgy? I think not. I bet we would find that, despite our bravado, we're all a little tentative when it comes to sex. Not just how to have it, but giving language to our deepest desires, longings, fears, conditioning, and insecurities. We do locker room talk with ease, but how easily do we express ourselves honestly and vulnerably? Fear drives most of our sexual behavior, but only because we've yet to take off the mask. The moment we do, we'll realize that we're all in the same boat. Everyone has some fear when it comes to sex.

My journey into sex began with fear. I was scared to talk to the people in my life about my sexual thoughts, feelings, and experiences. I thought I'd be looked at funny, judged, or made out to be some kind of freak. At such a sensitive time, all I really needed was someone to listen, someone to understand, and someone to hold space for all of my unanswered questions that I was too afraid to ask. While much has changed since then, since we first innocently discovered our sexuality, our fear of sex has not. Culturally, sex is still considered taboo. When I casually ask someone about their sex life, which I habitually do, I often see their butt cheeks clench. The discomfort is palpable. Sex is the one thing we all do that nobody wants to talk about, because talking about sex means you're "raunchy" or "dirty," but I assure you there's a way to talk about sex that isn't.

In order to transform our fear around sex, we're going to have to talk about it. We're going to have to come out of the sexual closet, so to speak. Not from a wounded place, but from a human place. From a place of honor, respect, honesty, and vulnerability. This doesn't mean everyone needs to get on the same page in terms of what's sexually "appropriate" and what's not. The goal isn't to universalize the experience. The goal is to liberate the fear that's been ingrained in us and do so in a way that protects everyone involved. We do that by creating containers; a safe, trustworthy, and reliable space where people can come together and share themselves vulnerably, while honoring the boundaries of the space.

As mind-blowing as I can make it sound, sex alone is no guarantee for transcendence. Two people must make themselves raw and vulnerable before one another in order to touch the higher realms of sex. One thing is for certain, true transcendence can never be had where love is withheld, and love is withheld anytime we engage in sexual activity from a place of fear. Even the slightest worry about the size of our penis or how long we'll last is enough to have us unintentionally withhold our love. There's a very fine line between sex that harms and sex that heals. Sex that harms is rooted in fear, and sex that heals is rooted in love.

Healing sex doesn't happen without our willingness to be real, raw, and vulnerable with each other. This doesn't mean we're not allowed to feel fear. It simply means coming clean with our fear as to not withhold love. This requires relational maturity, which presupposes a relationship, actually knowing somebody enough to trust them with your body, your mind, your heart, and your spirit. Our first and most important relationship is the one we have with ourselves. How well do we really know ourselves sexually? Have we asked ourselves the questions: what's right for me? What feels good to me? What doesn't feel good? How do I like to be talked to, interacted with, touched? What are my boundaries? What are my desires? How do I want to feel in this space?

These questions and questions like them are fundamental for exploring our unique sexual expression, as well as the kind of sex that feels most genuine for us. Doctors and researchers have found that most women first learn about sex from their initial relationships with men, boys who ninety-nine percent of the time learn about sex through porn. That means most women, at least since the dawn of the Internet, have been gaining their sexual awareness through what we could consider secondhand porn. The only way of changing any of this is by closing our laptops and facing each other.

It's time for us to stop trying to figure it all out on our own. Despite our fears, we need to normalize the conversation about sex. Not in a demeaning way, but in a way that honors sex as sacred and honors our body as the temple for this sacred act. If we can't talk about it amongst ourselves, how are we ever going to support future generations in discerning what's right for them? How are they ever going to feel safe to open up and share their thoughts, feeling, and wonders about sex? It starts with us being intimately connected to ourselves, our body and our own sexuality. Again, not from a wounded place, from our heart.

Once you know what feels right for you, then you can authentically communicate that to your partner. If your partner is comfortable with what you've shared and carries the same perspective, the two of you can move forward. If your partner's not comfortable with what you've shared, then there's more for the two of you to explore with your communication before exploring each other physically. Regardless, every time we have sex there must be mutual consent, and genuine consent requires verbal communication. Yes means yes, no means no, and maybe means maybe; without coercion, force, pressure, or shame. There has to be a mutual understanding that we will never attempt to meet our own desires at the expense of our partner.

This is called discernment. It applies across the board, whether you're having sex with someone for the first time or making love with your wife of twenty years. We treat every time as if it's the first time. It's this level of physical, mental, and emotional maturity that allows us to protect each other in this space. The sex industry thrives off of exploiting human beings, but what we miss is how often we unintentionally exploit each other by not effectively communicating our boundaries, desires, expectations, and fears. Communication like this brings two people together from any background and makes them equals in this space. It equalizes their power. That way neither person is vulnerable to exploitation by the other, even if it's unintended.

Creating a sacred container essentially handles all of this. By container, I simply mean an intentional space where two people reside. It's an energetic space, not something you're going to find at Home Depot. The two people occupying this space have specific agreements and promises that they've committed to upholding with one another. These are what I like to call sacred contracts. Our contracts create the container. Ideally, the two people creating the contracts have chosen to join in union. I'm not trying to seem uptight here, I simply believe that this level of commitment is required to access the deepest levels of intimacy, and therefore, ecstasy. Commitment is the building block of safety. Without it, it's easy for us to tuck tail and run at the first sign of discomfort. Safety softens people and evokes love, and love is the difference between sex that harms and sex that heals. If you choose to engage sexually and you're not in union, the same principle applies.

These contracts obviously encompass more than just sex. They're our promises to one another; how we promise to treat one another, how we promise to be with one another, and how we promise to show up for one another, especially when times get tough. They're our commitments, to ourselves, to each other, and to the union itself. They're what we turn to, reflect upon, and remember when things aren't as peachy as they were in the beginning. Think of them as the lighthouse keeping us orientated at sea, protecting us from shipwreck. They're the words we offer to one another and request that we be held accountable to.

Our contracts create the container. Inside the container, two people are free to be exactly as they are, to express their hearts openly and honestly, and safely explore themselves and each other on a much deeper level. It has the opposite effect of what you might imagine. We usually associate contracts with a loss of freedom, limiting what we can and cannot do, putting a cap on us so to speak, but because we've taken the time to clarify what's important to us, we're free to play inside our well-defined, protective structure. Think of it like learning the rules of a sport. Once you learn the rules of basketball; what's a foul and what's not, what's out of bounds, and what's illegal, you're clear about the container called "basketball." Inside this container you can start to develop your skills and master your craft. You could be the best ball handler in the world, but if you keep stepping out of bounds because you're not clear on the boundaries of the court, you're not going to thrive competitively. You might have the natural ability, athleticism, and skill to play in the big leagues, but your inability to honor the rules of the game will keep you from excelling.

Creating a container is surprisingly simple. The first step is to set sacred space just as you would if you were going to make love. Before entering the space, make sure that each of you has a pen and some paper. Just like legally binding contracts, these contracts are to be documented on paper. Relax, breathe, eye gaze, and take some time to become fully present. When you're ready, begin writing. Some questions to contemplate while creating your sacred contracts are:

- What does my partner and this relationship mean to me?
- What are my deal breakers? My nonnegotiables?
- What are my promises to my partner?
- What are my promises to myself?
- What can I be counted on for? What can I not be counted on for?
- What purpose will this container serve?

All of these questions and whatever others come to you intuitively will allow you to intentionally explore your containers' boundaries. It will help you more clearly define who you are, what you stand for, and what's expected of you from your partner. Do not rush this. These contracts will be the foundation for your entire relationship, not only your sex life. Take your time. Give yourself the chance to explore everything. Make sure you take time to consider every area of your life including your work, health, family, finances, service, communities, etc. Remember, these are your agreements, your promises, and your commitments to yourself, your lover, and your union.

When you've had sufficient time and feel complete with the process, share your contracts out loud with one another. Read them to each other one at a time. As your partner reads her contract, be present to every word. Allow her commitments to you to penetrate your heart. Allow your emotions to rise to the surface without blocking them. This is not a time for "being strong." Pay special attention to what's important to her. As you read your contract, allow for the same. These contracts plant the seeds of love, respect, honor, adoration, devotion, and reverence into the soil of your union. It is one of the most intimate experiences you can share with another. Allow it to be that.

In the aftermath of sharing, consummate the contracts. Allow every spoken word, every promise, every commitment, to fuse the two of you together in union. If you're not quite to that point yet, to a place where you feel fully safe to be sexually intimate, that's okay. Consummate the contracts another way, in a way that feels right for you. It doesn't have to be sex. Do something that signifies you've received each other's commitments, you're honoring what's been created, and you're now integrating it. Maybe you eye gaze, maybe you hold each other close, whatever feels aligned for you. Just make sure you don't kill the vibe by suggesting something stupid like watching Netflix.

You'll find in the days and weeks that follow that you feel differently towards one another. You'll feel more confident, more intimate, more exhilarated, and somehow freer. Above all, you'll feel an overwhelming sense of safety from knowing exactly where you and your partner stand with one another. This will ignite passion in your love-making and deepen your experience of intimacy, expanding your capacity for co-creating love through sex.

The trust established through this practice will grant you better access to yourself; your vulnerabilities, your desires, your feelings, your fears, and anything else on your heart. Give voice to those things, for it will undoubtedly be a "turn on." Your trust in the container will also allow you to more easily surrender into love-making. You'll stop trying to get it right, perform, act all machismo, and think you know everything there is to know about pleasuring a woman. Instead, you'll allow her to be your guide in discovering what's best for her body.

All of this open communication takes away any unspoken

performance pressures, allowing you both to relax. The more relaxed you are, the more you'll receive. You also won't feel so self-conscious about the not so comfortable parts of love-making either. Because you're having sex that heals, expect to be emotional. Expect to have things rise to the surface to be released from your body. Expect the same from her body. Don't be surprised if that emotion is gratitude for having been chosen for such epic love.

If it gets too uncomfortable at any point, just pause for a moment and relax. In the midst of your love-making, hold each other as only lovers can; passionately, compassionately, vulnerably, and tenderly. You have now consciously signed up to go far beyond anything you've ever experienced. Sacred contracts provide us with the safety, trust, confidence, and clarity we need to fully open ourselves to all there is to receive from love-making. They're a gift we give to ourselves, our permission slip to open our heart in new and exhilarating ways.

The last thing I'll share here is that it's important to take into consideration the whole person with whom you're joining with in union. Let me explain. When we begin new relationships and create new containers, it's because we've fallen in love with a person for who they are now, not who they've been at some other point in their life. We all have a past. In terms of union and what can rise to the surface to be healed, it's important we take into consideration our partner's past, including the emotionally traumatic experiences that took place long before we arrived.

When our partner suddenly bursts into tears during the act of love-making, we might think it's weird, awkward, or have a mini internal freak out. Our mind might race trying to figure out what went wrong. Meanwhile our body tenses up and freezes. Remember, love-making isn't a mind thing. This isn't something to freak out about. It's simply something from the past rising to the surface to be healed. Without our contracts, we're liable to misunderstand these experiences and think something's wrong, either with the relationship itself or specifically with the love-making. Instead of leaning into what's surfacing, we'll likely lean out, mentally rationalizing that this isn't what's supposed to happen during sex.

I assure you, experiences like this are totally normal. Instead of something being wrong with the relationship or wrong with the sex, something is very right. The container itself is presenting us with the opportunity to heal. Make a note here, safe and trustworthy containers will intentionally bring up unresolved emotions for them to be witnessed, loved, and healed. This is because our physical bodies, for the first time in our lives, feel safe in the container to let go of what they've been holding onto. When we're aware of this, we can meet these experiences with grace, love, patience, and compassion, rather than panic or confusion. The union itself is inviting us to examine what's left for us to feel and heal, and it's each person's responsibility to look at what that is for them.

With contracts, two potentially opposing forces can come together and direct their energy towards healing the past, rather than reinforcing it. It's one of the many powerful things about establishing a safe and trustworthy container, and it goes both ways. Don't be surprised if you too revisit some things from your past. Our love-making is forwarding our healing. With our contracts in place, we can trust that we're safe to let go of what's no longer serving us.

Chapter 14

Releasing Shame

A close friend of mine listened to my podcast episode on sex a few months ago. After listening, he shared with me that the podcast had inspired him to have a conversation with his wife, one that he hadn't yet realized he needed to have. The topic of that conversation? Probably not what you're thinking. It wasn't that he wanted to try new things, spice up their sex life, or invite other people into the bedroom. On the contrary, it was how my friend felt about his sexual history. He confessed to me that the immature decisions and promiscuity of his sexual past had him feeling like "damaged goods" for his wife. Now here's a guy who's the epitome of vitality, a devoted husband, loving father, and inspiring friend. Looking at him, you would have never known he felt this way. Someone so loving and mature, it was hard to imagine him having anything to be ashamed of, let alone something to do with sex.

As I said before, we all have a past, and for many of us, our sexual history is not necessarily something we're proud of. For my friend, he desired to come clean with his wife about an element of his past that he still carried shame around. His love for her means so much to him that he felt ashamed about the way he had shared his body with other women before coming into union with her. He felt tainted, used, dirty, and therefore lacking the same purity he witnessed in her. Being the man that he is, he did have that courageous conversation with his wife. In it, he shared his heart, revealed his shame, and successfully released it by talking about it openly, honestly, and vulnerably. To his surprise, this created a depth of intimacy between him and his wife that they had both been longing for. To my surprise, he was writing to me to say thank you.

We all have a part of our sexual past that we feel ashamed of, at least until we come forward with it like my friend did. For me, it was the fact that I had gotten drunk, blacked out, and cheated on my last romantic partner preceding my beloved Makenzie. What was eating me alive was the fact that I hadn't shared that with anyone, not even my ex. I remember when it happened. I woke up next to a stranger laying naked in my bed, a woman that had just started dating my roommate at the time. Confused, hungover, and immediately devastated, it wasn't until my roommate debriefed me on the events of the evening prior that I got the full picture.

Not only had I hooked up with the girl he was dating, but I had also cheated on my girlfriend with whom I was in a long distance relationship, effectively damaging two meaningful relationships in one blow. It just so happened that I was flying to see my girlfriend the following weekend. My chance to come clean, be a man, and be honest about what had happened. I remember feeling so heavy with guilt and shame. I must have cried the entire four-hour flight over. I knew I needed to tell her the truth and let the rest go however it was meant to go, but when the time came for me to reveal what happened, I couldn't do it.

I couldn't bring myself to break her heart, end our relationship, and destroy my reputation over something that I couldn't even remember. My self-preservation got the best of me. Instead, I ate the truth, and it ate at me from that moment forward. Eventually this relationship did end. I somehow managed to escape with my reputation intact, even though I couldn't escape my feelings of guilt and shame. The experience haunted me, hung over me like a dark cloud.

Coming into union with my beloved quickly forced my little secret right back up to the surface. I had already felt like a total fraud, but to look into my beloved's eyes and withhold anything from her felt criminal. Did I dare try to build the relationship of my dreams on top of a lie? I was so afraid to tell her, terrified that she would think less of me, better yet not want to be with me at all. It got to the point where I simply couldn't live with myself anymore. My secret was eating me alive. So, I came clean. I broke down and told her the truth, despite my fear of what would happen next.

Turns out, for her, it wasn't such a big deal. I think she responded with something along the lines of, "Really? That's it? I thought for sure you were going to say something way worse than that." She went on to share how she had cheated, especially emotionally, in a number of her past relationships. We came to the conclusion that none of that really mattered anymore, and that the guilt and shame I was still carrying really wasn't serving me. In fact, because it was having me beat myself up over the past, it was keeping me from seeing the man that my beloved saw when she looked at me. I had learned my lesson and already caused myself enough grief muddling over the past. Yes, I had cheated. Yes, I had withheld the truth, but that didn't mean I was a bad person. It simply meant that I was human, that I made a mistake.

Nothing is so bad that it cannot be forgiven, and the time had come for me to forgive myself. Not that we shouldn't be responsible for our actions. Responsibility is much different than shame. Responsibility is taking ownership of what happened. Shame is letting the events of the past linger like a dark shadow over the present and future. Shame is believing we're unworthy of love and respect because of our thoughts, feelings, and actions. What happened, happened. I cheated. What didn't need to happen was for me to let my past torment me any further. I didn't need to let it destroy the possibility of a beautiful relationship with my beloved.

Coming clean with my beloved about my shameful secret not only brought me a deep sense of relief, but also strengthened our bond. I had now shared something with her that I had never shared with anyone, and she was grateful for my honesty. Her compassion for me invited me into compassion for myself, which only brought me closer to my center. If I could share my deepest, darkest secrets and still be loved for who I really was underneath my shame, then I was finally free to be the real me, something I had been working towards my entire life. This experience revealed to me that there was nothing I couldn't share. My sharing, as difficult as it felt for me at times, was actually desired. It created intimacy instead of the disappointment I anticipated. Revealing those scary parts of my past had me feel deeply seen, known, accepted, and loved for who I am, despite my past. This in turn finally allowed me to start loving myself.

At that point, I just assumed that was everything. It wasn't until I hosted my first ever HuMANity one-on-one session that something again rose to the surface. In my conversation with a client, where he was revealing to me something that he had never shared with anyone, a part of his sexual past that he was deeply ashamed of, I had a spontaneous memory of a sexual trauma from my past. It didn't involve anyone else and nothing inappropriate had been done to me. Instead, it was something I had done in private, when no one else was around.

Shortly after puberty, I was so curious and desperate to know what sex felt like, so that I could one day be ready for the real thing, that I tried to penetrate our family dog. I was a teenager when it happened, but since that day, I had never shared that with anyone. I was too ashamed. I was certain that it was the one thing that would have others look at me like some kind of monster, an experience I would undoubtedly take to my grave. It was also the thing that had me feel the most unworthy of love. It kept me from receiving people's adoration, the voice inside my head saying, "if you only knew who I really was, what I had done, you wouldn't love me the way you do."

Again, here was my chance to open up, let someone in, and

let go of the shame I had been holding onto for nearly twenty years now. This time, much more confident about the safety of our container, I went upstairs right after the call, sat my beloved down, and shared with her what I had experienced so many years ago. I balled my eyes out as she held my inner innocence. Again, she met my share with a compassionate share of her own, something from her sexual past that she too had never shared with anyone. In the aftermath of intimacy, we cried in each other's arms. A burden had been lifted. The sexual shame of my past had been brought to love once more.

I ended up sharing this experience with a group of close brothers in the next HuMANity Huddle session that I held less than a week later. They too met my experience with compassion and opened up about their own sexual trauma. I realized something in those moments, more than at any other point in my life. We all have something from our past, a sexual experience of some kind that we're ashamed of. Every single one of us longs to be free from our shame, but we're all scared to give our shame a voice. We all think that what we did or what happened to us could never be met with compassion. We're afraid of what others might think, what they might say, how our reputation might be damaged, all because we're already directing that kind of hatred towards ourselves. We're afraid people will see us the way we already see ourselves. The longer we remain silent, the more our shame erodes our sense of self-love and self-respect, but it doesn't have to be this way.

Truth is, we're all safer than we've ever been to open up and share about our shameful experiences. It's our freedom that's on the line if we don't. We get to choose whether our shame erodes our sense of self or connects us intimately with others. We get to choose whether or not our shame hovers over us like a dark cloud, or whether or not we bravely release it once and for all. It will require bravery, make no mistake. I can't promise you that the people in your life will love and respect you more for your honesty. They may not, but I can promise that you will. This is about your relationship with yourself, not anyone else. This is about you being whole and complete with yourself before ever extending your hand towards another. If some people in your life can't accept the actions of your past, then those probably aren't your people. You'll be doing yourself a favor by only surrounding yourself with those people that can love and accept you for who you are, all of who you are.

My question for you is this: where are you still holding onto the sexual shame of your past? Where are you still hiding something that you think will destroy you if you reveal it? It's often much easier for us to forgive those that have sexually traumatized us than it is for us to forgive ourselves for what we've done or allowed to happen. I'm not saying you have to open up and share your history with the world. I'm saying you'll find great relief in sharing it with someone you trust, inside of a container you trust. It's worth at least taking a good clean look for yourself.

We open our hearts to forgiveness by being brave enough to share. As much as this creates intimacy and freedom in our union, more importantly, it creates intimacy and freedom with ourselves. It's our fear that keeps us from liberation; fear of being rejected, fear of being cast out, fear of being ostracized, and fear of being condemned. In reality, those fears aren't about other people. They're a reflection of how we're already treating ourselves inside.

Our past sexual traumas are already a part of us that we internally condemn. For so many of us, these sexual experiences happened while we were still in our innocence. Many of us were very young when we first adopted shame, and it's our innocence that continues to suffer when we hold onto it. Be brave and thorough. Create sacred space and sit your partner down before you share. Allow yourself to be caught and received in your innocence, even if it was something that you did rather than something that was done to you.

Often relationships plateau because two people are unwilling to go to these depths with one another. It's only ever fear that keeps us from going there. I promise you, whatever it is, it's not beyond the reach of forgiveness and grace. Not to say that there won't be any real-life consequences of coming clean. There may be an impact for you to be radically responsible for, but there's also being responsible for the impact that our shame has on us. I assure you, that impact is greater than you realize. More than likely, you will find, just like I did, that your sharing evokes a similar share from your partner, in which case, you'll get to be responsible for the depth of intimacy that gets created in your union.

As men, this is space we can hold for each other as well. In the men's circles I've held, like the one I already mentioned, I've witnessed men be incredibly generous and compassionate with one another. We understand each other. We get what it's like to be people with similar conditioning. We understand each other's struggles, but also our commitment to our word, to who we say we're committed to being. Accountability is the key. Women are incredible at holding men accountable to their word, especially as it relates to sex. As men, we sometimes let each other off the hook. There's still this strong desire amongst us to want to be one of the guys and fit in. I know I'm always having to check myself on it in these spaces. I'm having to make sure I'm holding to my truth rather than letting it slide for the sake of getting along.

Any time I've opened up my heart and let myself be seen by other men it's been incredibly healing. Any time I've gone there and revealed my shame, I've been met with compassion and understanding. Going first in this way helps other men get real about their own shame. We have to remember that we're all in the same boat together. No more suffering in silence. We can hold this space of safety for one another. I've done this countless times for my brothers and received the same graciousness from them in return. Regardless, there will come a time for us to share ourselves in this way with our partner. Don't bypass this piece because of your distrust in women. It's required for the healing work we're here to do together.

Our sexual shame impacts us primarily through our silence. When we open up and share within the safety of a well-established container, we realize more often than not that just about everybody else is in the same boat as us. Whether we are embarrassed by how many times we've carelessly given our body away or hesitant to admit how inexperienced we are, we need to open up and share our shame. Shame is contagious, and right now just about everyone is infected. The remedy is truth, vulnerability, honesty, and compassion.

Sometimes it's not pretty. Sometimes we need to go to some dark places to expose our shame, but we must go there. Otherwise, the same shame that's in us today will infect our children tomorrow. They need to know that babies aren't delivered by storks and that sexuality is not the absence of morality. Our liberation from our sexual shame directly impacts our ability to positively educate our children. We must free ourselves first. Put the oxygen mask on ourselves first. We can't expect our children to lead us in a conversation about sex. We also can't continue avoiding it. We must use our words, voice our truth, and be honest about the things we're unsure of.

How we talk about sex has long and powerful implications. We needn't look any further than our own life experience to recognize that. We are the product of a generation that was, for the most part, afraid to talk about sex. Will we continue this legacy? The choice is ours and ours alone. There's no cavalry coming to save us. It either ends with us or gets passed on to our children. Future generations are counting on us. Let's not disappoint.

Chapter 15

Setting Sacred Space

Setting sacred space is essential for experiencing the sacredness of sex. It's like foreplay for the spiritual dimension. Just as we wouldn't expect to penetrate our woman without first invoking her heart, we also wouldn't expect to experience the sacredness of sex without first invoking the sacredness of the space. The intention with which we set sacred space directly impacts our experience of love-making.

Real love-making is a ceremony. In ceremony we perform ritual acts. Every act carries an intention, has a purpose. In love-making, we're courting the divine. Our intention is to unite our humanity with our divinity. Actualizing this intention requires preparation, introspection, time, space setting, and many other important things. We're not only merging our physical bodies in the act of love-making, we're also merging our energy bodies. Our two separate energy bodies are coming together to become one shared whole. This shared field strips us of any inauthenticity, shucks us like a cob of corn. What isn't discarded is alchemized into the union and becomes a part of who we are.

In preparing for love-making, it's important that we check in and get connected to our physical body. We can do this by breathing intentionally. With each breath, we scan our physical body for anything we wouldn't want to bring with us into the love-making space. Are we holding tension? Are we anxious? Is our mind at peace or is it everywhere other than this present moment? Are we feeling nourished enough to enter this space and hold the vibration it requires? Or do we feel depleted, tired, in need of nourishment? All of these questions and whatever other questions come to you intuitively serve us in returning our awareness to our physical body, and therefore, the present moment.

Sometimes the answer to these questions can be something along the lines of, "no, I don't feel energized enough for love-making. In this moment, my body needs rest." It's okay to be a no. It's a simple matter of integrity that we honor our body's needs prior to love-making. If I'm bloated, exhausted, constipated, and irritable, then my body is certainly not going to be a full "fuck yes" to love-making. In the past, I might have ignored this and pretended I was a full "yes" to avoid my beloved feeling rejected or me feeling less manly, since being a man means being ready to jump in the sack at any moment.

Anytime my body was a "no" but I said "yes," something big always came up. My physical discomfort would keep me from being all in and my beloved, being the incredibly intuitive woman she is, would feel that. I'll sum it up by saying, it usually didn't go well. We would of course navigate through it together, but the situation became more complex than it ever needed to be. These days, I'm not a full "yes" to love-making unless I know my body is ready to go the energetic distance, to surrender fully into the ceremony of love-making. Anything less just isn't worth it to me.

Even when I'm exhausted, I could still get aroused, penetrate her, and release, but the physical act alone pales in comparison to the real deal. The difference between the two is a simple matter of integrity. That's not to say there aren't things we can do to help our body become a "yes," like go to the bathroom, breathe, take a few moments of stillness, ground outside, go on a walk, brush our teeth, shower, or get nourished with food or water. It's simply means that our body will always be our guide for whether or not to initiate love-making. When our body is a "yes," there are a few integral things we can do to properly prepare for ceremony.

The first thing is getting our love-making scheduled on the calendar. I know, it seems like this would suck the excitement right out of the occasion, but if you're somebody that's up to anything in life, then you probably don't have a lot of extra time laying around just waiting to be filled. Set a nonnegotiable time for when you and your beloved will come together to make love. Yes, actually put it in your calendar. That way you're prioritizing love-making. This allows us to know when the ceremony of love-making is going to begin and gives us ample time to prepare. For example, if I know that my beloved and I are making love at 6:00 p.m., then by 5:00 p.m., I'm already tuning into my body. I'm starting my intentional breathing, even if I'm still working. I'm relaxing any tension and starting to contemplate what I want to co-create with her.

Having it scheduled also reminds me not to have a three-course meal at 5:30 p.m. Instead, I'll fast, hydrate my body, or snack if I'm hungry. Sometimes I'll stretch, put my bare feet on the ground, or take a shower. No matter what, I always make sure to get off technology at least twenty minutes beforehand and do some intentional breathing. For me, this immediately connects me with my sex energy, gives me a pulse for where it's at. It prepares my awareness to channel it consciously.

No matter how you choose to prepare your body, mind, and heart for love-making, knowing when to start the preparation process is essential. It's not practical to expect that we or our beloved should be ready to transition at the drop of a dime from whatever we were doing to the space of love-making, especially when our days are mostly filled with work, stress, technology, physical inactivity, and excessive mental stimulation. There needs to be a period of time prior to love-making for us come back to ourselves before offering ourselves to our partner. That way we can be certain that we're bringing our best-self forward into this space.

At first, I had a lot of resistance to this because it seemed to eliminate the possibility of spontaneity, those times I'm inspired to passionately disrobe my beloved and ravish her on the spot. It seemed like I would have to forfeit that element of our relationship, but boy was I wrong. By prioritizing this time to prepare for love-making, not only did we deepen our capacity for intimacy by making sure we had no time constraints, but the love-making became so consistently "out of this world" that the frequency of these "spontaneous ravishings" increased. In a way, it's like the love-making never ended. We were so connected to the depths of intimacy awaiting us just beyond our ordinary, everyday interactions, that we ended up in a consistent state of foreplay.

Another important point to emphasize here is that the female body normally opens to love-making much more slowly than the male body. This is not always the case, but most of the time it reigns true. As men, we can become aroused at the drop of a dime. Women are less singularly focused. What arouses them is often much different than what arouses us. Think sensuality rather than sexuality. Sensuality obviously has everything to do with the senses, and there are many; taste, touch, sight, smell, hearing, balance, temperature, proprioception, etc.

It can take time for a woman to transition from whatever hat she's wearing to "romantic lover." It can take time for her to reconnect with her sensual body. This is especially true for women who wear many hats: wife, mother, friend, daughter, boss, leader, caretaker, etc. They're the opposite of singularly focused, usually connected to all things at once. As a man, we can certainly aid her in making this transition. Something as simple as cleaning the house or cleaning the room in which we're about to make love in goes a long way in terms of giving her one less thing to think about.

Sometimes there's much to divulge verbally before our bodies start talking. Inviting her to share might help empty her internal space a bit. A woman can feel any number of emotions before brushing her teeth in the morning. Sometimes it's good to give those emotions some space to come out before love-making.

This can be as simple as asking her, "how's your heart?" Then zipping our lips and intentionally listening. You feeling into her in this way, showing her that you care for her emotions, will undoubtedly be a turn on for her. Ninety percent of the time she needs to be opened slowly, the other ten percent she's ready to go just like you are. So, take your time. Be romantic. Compliment her on her appearance, acknowledge her for her work, tidy up your sacred space, put on some music, set out some flowers, delight her senses. Court the romantic lover in her and witness as she steps forward to reembrace her sensuality.

The second thing we can do to properly prepare for love-making is set sacred space. By this, I mean clean up both the physical and energetic space within which we're going to make love. Pick up the clothes, make the bed, and declutter the clutter. Burn some sage or Palo Santo as you energetically clear any and all remaining work energy, stress, or emotional density from the day. Get rid of the distractions. Turn off the TV, switch your phones to airplane mode, dim the lights, and light some candles. Close the windows if it's noisy outside and play some serenading music. Say an intentional blessing over the space, either in your mind or out loud. I recommend out loud. Welcome in your spirit team and divine helpers; your higher-self, spirit guides, angels, archangels, teachers, etc. Allow them to bless the space with their presence. Ask them for assistance with cleansing and clearing the energy of the space until all that remains is the highest vibration of unconditional love. This process looks different for every couple and includes whatever things you feel are sacred. Your process may be very different from what I've described. Discover what works for you, what heightens your senses, invokes the sacred, and creates an environment of love and safety.

Invite your awareness powerfully into the present moment and consciously create your intentions for love-making. No intention is too large or too small. Sit face to face with your beloved before initiating anything physical. Look into her eyes and fully receive her, witness her brilliance, allow yourself to be moved by her magnificence. When you're both ready, share your intentions out loud, one person at a time. These intentions are quite literally what you are committed to co-creating with this love-making session.

What is it that you're desiring to conceive and birth into the world? What are you desiring to devote the potency of your love-making towards? Something for yourself, your beloved, your union, your family, your businesses, creative projects, communities, something for the entire world? Place your hand over your beloved's heart and breathe with her, inhaling and exhaling as her breath rises and falls. Let your heart be penetrated by your love for her as well as her love for you. Allow that feeling to permeate every cell of your body.

Now you've arrived. You've intentionally entered into the sacred space of loving-making, fully prepared and ready to merge with your beloved. While your path may not identically mirror mine, you've taken all the steps to invoke the sacredness of the space. Now... let go. Let go of everything you think you know about sex and let your spirit move you. Allow your movements to be completely intuitive. You're in a divine dance of ecstasy with no foreseeable end in sight, surrender. It could go on forever as far as you're concerned. Let go. Let your higher-self move your body.

There's no rush here, nowhere to go, nowhere else to be, nothing to get to. In this space five minutes can feel like three hours and three hours like five minutes. Time and space become irrelevant because you're transcending both. Breathe, relax, receive, and allow your creative energy to circulate. The more relaxed you are the more you will receive, the greater the pleasure will be. Allow for everything. Trust everything; every sensation, every feeling, every emotion, every intuitive nudge. There have been times when I have emotionally released in this space, times when I've suddenly burst into tears. There have been times when my beloved has burst into tears. There have been times where I've giggled like a child, laughed out loud, and paused to share something with my beloved while still resting inside her. Nothing is off limits. When we set sacred space everything that unfolds inside that space is sacred, perfect, and exactly as it is meant to be. Everything is unfolding in its own divine timing. Trust it. Trust in your own ability to trust it.

Sometimes our higher-selves will reveal a vision to us. Sometimes our bodies will recognize the safety of the container and go into a healing process. Don't try to make logical sense of it all. It's deep, expansive, and life-altering work, far beyond the capacity of the mind. Whatever shows up in this love-making space, allow for it. Remember to breathe and circulate your sex energy throughout your entire body. We have talked about lingam massage and your preparation for this moment. You have the skills to pull back your energy if it starts to feel too intense, like you might release before you're ready. Come back to your breath and intentionally relax your body. Visualize the energy moving from the tip of your lingam back into your body where it can once again disperse itself inwardly. This is a learned skill that's well worth practicing.

If you're guided to move faster and with greater intensity, do so, but also allow for slower movements with greater sensitivity. A woman's body is capable of fully receiving both, and both can be equally pleasurable for her. You don't need to rush her to orgasm. Her body was brilliantly designed to experience orgasm long before she ever reaches climax. When both of your hearts are open, your hearts will orgasm together completely independent of your sex organs. Once you experience this, it will forever alter your reality around love-making.

An orgasming heart has the ability to extend far beyond the act of love-making. You might find that you're not even doing anything sexual when you experience it. You could be washing the dishes in your kitchen when you're suddenly overcome by how grateful you are for your life. You could watch your beloved read a book or write in her journal and feel completely overwhelmed by her radiance. You could hear a child laughing and immediately know nothing but joy. When the heart orgasms, we experience ourselves at one with life. In those moments, we're no longer our ego, our identity, or our personality. We are love itself.

You don't need to be in divine union to experience this love. You just need to devote the same level of intention you would towards your external beloved inward towards your internal beloved, your higher-self. It's not something to feel sheepish about either. The deepest truth is that we are all, in essence, our own beloved. When we make love to another, we are really making love to another aspect of ourselves. We're touching a love that lives inside all of us. The same thing is happening when you massage yourself.

Every living thing on our planet is impacted by the love we do or don't create in love-making. Make it count. Let's make sure the legacy we leave as men and fathers for the generations to come is one of unconditional love, including unconditional self-love.

As a recap, here are the general guidelines to follow when setting sacred space for love-making:

- Schedule it. Make it a date!
- Prepare your body
- Set sacred space
- Create and share your intentions
- Be fully present and aware
- Scan and relax your body
- Breathe deeply and slowly
- Enter her slowly, without force
- Move intuitively

- Allow the excitement to build and relax, build and relax
- Keep your eyes open, maintain eye contact
- Don't be afraid to pause
- Remember, the goal is to be goalless. Let that shit go.
- Have fun

As with anything, what's the point of love-making if we're not having fun? Be willing to laugh at yourself and let things go like water off a duck's back. Presence and awareness during love-making creates and nourishes connection. Setting sacred space helps us experience love-making for what it is, a gift. It's our gift to ourselves, each other, and the rest of the world, something we're here to give wholeheartedly.

Chapter 16

The Willingness to Give

This dissolution of self into the oneness of all that is, is an experience that we as men are designed to offer our beloved in this sacred space of love-making. Through the safety of our consciously created container, the intentions we set prior to love-making, the way we set sacred space, and the way we surrender during the act, our love-making becomes a vessel for the divine. We penetrate our beloved with the love of the divine. In witnessing her receive, we receive. Our hearts are filled by witnessing our beloved open, step through those ecstatic gates, and receive divine nourishment. Witnessing her is like drinking the divine nectar of the goddess. It fulfills a part of us like nothing else can. It's also one of the most powerful ways that we can nourish and support our beloved.

Nothing compares to love-making in terms of giving and receiving love. Where women typically need to be physically, mentally, and emotionally nurtured in order to feel safe to open, men often need love-making to feel fully safe to open their hearts. Love-making is a powerful means through which men feel emotionally connected to their lovers, and therefore themselves; a space where all the normal barriers to receiving love more easily come down. For me, love-making is one of the most powerful ways in which I experience intimacy with my beloved. When we make love, my heart opens, my body relaxes, my mind dissolves, and I feel the power and potency of our connection.

As I look into my beloved's eyes, any resistance I have to receiving love dissolves. I find myself deeply immersed in a full body/heart orgasm. The apparent separation between her body and mine disappears and all that remains is an undeniable experience of oneness. There is only us and a feeling of unity that dissolves any sense of space and time and our apparent differences in anatomy. While it has taken years of practice, years of learning to surrender and let go into this experience, allowing the magic to happen all on its own, at this point, this oneness is something I experience with my beloved every time we make love. For me, it's one of life's greatest blessings, as well as one of life's greatest mysteries.

As men, being fully immersed with our beloved in this experience of oneness is something that we're absolutely capable of creating. The way we set sacred space is a signal to our partner that she's safe to open to this deep dive. Sex is by no means the only way of accessing this experience of oneness. Breathwork, extensive meditation, yogic practices, plant medicines; they all offer us the opportunity to reach these ecstatic states, each one taking its own unique route to get there, each one requiring something different from us. Where some require exertion, I have found this pathway to be one of surrender, a letting go of what we're not to make way for all that we are.

If we're capable of it, why not allow our love-making to be an all-inclusive vacation from the density of the world? Why not have our love-making be an experience that leaves us more intimately connected with who we really are, even if only for a little while? One of the many gifts of this space is that it's an opportunity to let go into this oneness. Yes, simple things like letting go of our day, our troubles, what worries us and what doesn't, but also bigger things like our ego, our identity, our personality, and our perspectives; all the things we think make us who we are. Not to escape them, but to remember that they're more like an outfit we wear rather than who we really are. We can change our outfit at any time, but we cannot change our fundamental interconnectedness.

Just because this experience is ecstatic doesn't mean we'll easily receive it. Love like this will bring us up against all of our barriers to receiving; things like unworthiness, shame, embarrassment, judgment, self-criticism, and the all-around physical discomfort associated with receiving. That's our practice, receiving, for both men and women alike. If we can surrender into it here, in the safety of our container, then we can surrender into it elsewhere. Our container is where we practice. Receiving is the spiritual work of the twenty-first century. We've built a lot of barriers to letting the "good stuff" in. This is one space we can utilize to start removing those barriers. We can start healing what's in the way of our ability to receive love.

We can take our giving and receiving into the physical particulars of love-making too. Orgasm is a powerful means through which our beloved experiences her sensuality, her sexuality, her femininity, and her goddess archetype. It connects her intimately with her body, the source of her greatest creativity, connectivity, intuition, and wisdom. Because the female body works so differently than the male body, at least in terms of sexual pleasure and orgasm, it's important for us to give pleasure in a way that our beloved can receive it. This is very specific to our partner, how her body works, what she prefers, and what feels good to her.

For the man, this means making the time to become familiar with our partner's body and the way in which it receives pleasure. Yes, this means having open conversations about it, looking at her body, exploring her female anatomy, and asking her some good question like, "does that feel good? What about this?" It may seem awkward at first, and of course our sexual interactions won't always contain such open, explorative dialogue, but it's important to explore, nevertheless.

Dialogue like this will provide you with important information on what feels right for her, that way when the two of you are well on your way to those ecstatic gates, you won't be stuck up in your head wondering if she's really feeling it or not.

Instead, you'll have peace of mind knowing that if she needs something different, she'll let you know. This way you'll be free to give to her and receive for yourself the one of a kind feeling that comes from having thoroughly satisfied your lover.

This means no more faking it! No more pretending she's feeling pleasure if the truth is, she's not. This doesn't mean we'll be perfect. We won't always ring her bells and blow her whistles just right. It's not about that. It's about taking the ego out of love-making and realizing that just as our beloved has unique ways in which she receives love (words of affirmation, time spent, thoughtful gifts, physical touch, etc.), she also has unique ways in which she receives pleasure. Knowing those ways increases our odds of delivering pleasure and satisfaction in our love-making.

Many women can't orgasm through vaginal penetration alone. For those women, other means are required to reach their peaks of pleasure. Not to emphasize orgasm as the point or purpose of love-making. We're simply exploring it here because it's obviously an inherent part of sex, and one part in particular that's capable of delivering immense pleasure to the woman we love. Like I said before, there's no rush in love-making. Sex is so much more than just a sprint to orgasm. Knowing your beloved's body and how it works will allow you to better pleasure her in a way that she can receive. Sex, or what I am calling love-making, is defined in literature and scholarly texts as penetration. The first statement in this paragraph is evidence enough that this definition clearly doesn't work for everyone.

I've elaborated a lot already on the spiritual aspects of love-making because knowing them is so important. Now that we've laid the proper groundwork for love-making, we are ready to dive into the next layer. I believe the conversation about female genitalia is one that should be normalized between lovers. In the little research I did creating this book, I discovered that the barrage of sexual shame directed towards women, primarily from men, is what has kept many women from sexually exploring their body. Many women, just like the men interacting with them, have little to no understanding of their female anatomy, including how it all works. The fear of being publicly ridiculed, shamed, or openly labeled a slut, tramp, whore, nympho, seductress, or any other derogatory term, has unfortunately kept many women from shamelessly exploring their body's full capacity for receiving pleasure. We've all played our part in this.

The truth is, most men don't actually want a sexually empowered woman because the idea of feeling sexually inferior to a woman is so debilitating to the male ego. Most men would rather jump off a bridge than have a woman guide them through providing her pleasure. In more cases than not, our fear of embarrassment or rejection stops us from being properly educated by our lovers. It's time we go beyond the limitations of our masculine ego and discover, maybe for the first time, what actually brings pleasure to our beloved. It goes without saying that this is an inherently sensitive topic for both sexes, one that I'm sure we all desire to feel a little bit more confident about. Lucky for us, our exploration of sexual pleasure is something we get to do inside of our co-created container. That safety is what will result in a very special kind of sexual experience.

The first thing to recognize here is that pleasure doesn't require two people being naked together. There are many ways to pleasure a woman long before taking her clothes off, let alone making contact with her body. The first is quite simple but often overlooked. Men are guilty of trying to play it cool when it comes to sex; sitting back, waiting, thinking that their handsome looks, attractive body, and laid-back demeanor is something like a dinner bell for their beloved's sexual appetite. I'm guilty of this as well. For years I thought this "too cool for school" attitude was irresistible to the opposite sex. Sit back, play it cool, don't show my cards, and let them come to me. Am I Right? You too? This stuck with me all the way up into my relationship with my beloved. I used to sit back, be passive, and do my best to play it cool while expecting her to become spontaneously aroused by my ever-obvious masculine mojo (that's me making fun of myself if you can't tell).

I expected her to come onto me. Sometimes she did, especially early on in our relationship when we were flying high on infatuation. However, for the long term, if I wanted to enjoy consistent love-making with my beloved, then I needed to assume my rightful role as the initiator. Being the initiator means taking full responsibility for the sexual activity or inactivity of the relationship. It means it's on us to create the structure required for both lovers to thrive. That means playing the primary role in scheduling love-making, setting sacred space, initiating intention setting, and creating emotional intimacy by asking things like, "how's your heart?"

For a long time, I didn't do this. Instead, I elected to harbor resentment anytime we weren't making love as often as I wanted. My ego was like, "WTF? Why does this person not want to have sex with me? I'm sexy. I'm heart-centered. I'm emotionally intelligent. WTF? I deserve better. I deserve to be desired the same way I desire her, blah, blah, blah." It was ugly, and honestly, a real sore spot for us for a while. My beloved was obviously hurt and confused by my resentment. Like, "bro, WTF? If you want more love-making, then man up and make it happen."

As you can imagine, my ego didn't like hearing that. With all due respect, she was right. I was being passive, letting all my immature, past-based conditioning get the best of me. So, I essentially reached down in my pants and had a rather unpleasant "come to Jesus" talk with myself. I decided right then and there that I was going to stop being such a victim and take on full responsibility for creating intimacy in our union. I know, many of you are going to hate me for being the whistle blower on this, but it's time. The good news is that you already know how to initiate. I already elaborated on that in the last chapter. Most of the "how-to" aspect is already handled.

How else can you pleasure your woman before penetrating her physically? You can talk to her. I'm not talking *Fifty Shades of Gray* here. I'm talking better than that; real, intimate, heart-centered sharing. Like how in love with her you are, how lucky you feel to be her man, and how grateful you are to get to be with her this way. I typically fall on the reserved side when it comes to verbal expression, but I tell you what, in the heat of the moment, I'm using my words just as much as my body to prepare my beloved to receive me. I learned to be this way because "words of affirmation" just so happens to be my beloved's primary love language. It's how she receives love. That may be different for your beloved, but that's up to you to figure out.

As I'm verbally expressing my love, I'm also massaging her body with my hands. I'm grabbing her hips, massaging her thighs, gripping the back of her neck and shoulders, scratching the top of her head with my fingertips, all the while intentionally circulating my sex energy through her body. I'm using my chin to massage the tense muscles of her neck, making my way up and down her sternocleidomastoid, working the muscle belly from origin to insertion. All of this happens intuitively when I surrender.

Eyes open, bodies merged, we're already locked into the sensation of orgasms long before penetration. I contemplated giving a template for pleasuring a woman, but every woman is so different that it just wouldn't work. Instead, I encourage you to be less interested in your own pleasure and more interested in understanding your woman's body. Communication is key, especially before being one hundred percent certain of what feels good to her. If she's not sure what feels good to her, be open to discovering it together.

Nothing quite compares to witnessing my beloved receive pleasure. There are times when I give purely for the pleasure I receive from witnessing her receive. Which brings up a valuable point. Just because the penetration portion of sex is over doesn't mean the love-making is complete. It's incredibly important to linger in this space. I love to tickle my beloved's back, gently graze her skin with my fingertips, let her head and torso rest against my body. Sometimes I continue on pleasuring her even after I've released. Other times we laugh, giggle, rest, sigh, and express our amazement. Sometimes we fall asleep together. Sometimes we express softly what we experienced; messages we heard, visions we received, any emotions we felt throughout the ceremony.

I personally love hearing about my beloved's experience because it makes me feel even more intimately connected to her. My point is, don't just break the space and rush off to whatever you were doing before you started making love. Rest and relax here. This post love-making time for cuddling, connection, rest, and sharing your heart is just as essential as setting sacred space. It's also where you build your energy body. It will fill your love cup for days, maybe even weeks. Do this and you'll find your mood is quite delightful, your demeanor positive, and your rapport with your beloved easy and graceful.

When we educate ourselves on what feels good for our beloved, we narrow the pleasure gap between men and women. The female body is miraculous in its ability to feel. She can experience the greatest heights of ecstasy in one moment followed by the deepest depths of despair in the next. Her capacity to receive pleasure is beyond anything anyone of us could imagine, which is precisely why it's so important to allow her to share with us what has her reach her heights. You may find that she has yet to explore this side of herself. Perfect, do it together. While you're doing it, be gracious, loving, sensitive, and kind. This can be such a sensitive topic but ultimately, it's one more thing that will bring the two of you closer together. When you're intimately connected to what brings your woman pleasure, it's kind of like having a secret superpower. You know you can please her, she knows you can please her, and the rest is just surrendering into how it plays out.

For us, we often dumb our pleasure down to stimulation and release, stimulation and release. The female body requires much more attention, much more intention, much more care. When we're willing to humble ourselves enough and set aside our ego's need to feel like sex's version of Muhamad Ali, we can learn what actually pleasures our beloved. This is where the adventure really begins. Mastering the physical side of sex allows us to more easily access the spiritual. We're free to float in this sacred space of oneness for as long as we're willing to tolerate it. It starts with our willingness to give, our willingness to trash everything we think we know about sex and pleasure and start from scratch, with our beloved as our guide. As always, let it be fun and playful.

Something to keep in mind. Nearly all of us had some kind of upbringing that made us believe sex was shameful. While we have long outgrown our shame-filled upbringing, our body still remembers. Our body still remembers all of the environmental imprinting it received during our first seven years of life. From an ancestral perspective, women throughout the course of history have had to be fearful of men's sex energy as it was often forced upon them. Because we're so physically different and because women throughout history were viewed as the property of men, subjects of lesser social value, ancestrally, women have had to fear being taken as sex objects against their will for as long as our history permits remembrance. This too is something the body remembers. Given how much this is still a part of our culture, don't be surprised if your woman doesn't quite feel fully safe to explore her sexuality. Remember the bigger picture. No more shaming her for this. As men, we can do our part in reconciling our ancestry and helping her feel physically safe again. Don't get frustrated. See the bigger picture. Be in it for the long-term and bear witness to her blossoming.

Chapter 17

Looking for Love in All the Wrong Places

I used to sleep with women to get high. I used to date women to get high. I didn't know it at the time. I simply thought that I was "in love." Relationship after relationship, in love and out of love, in love and out of love, like clockwork. In love while riding the cocktail of testosterone, phenylethylamine, norepinephrine, dopamine, oxytocin, serotonin, and endorphins pumping through my veins and very much out of love once those love chemicals wore off. I was an addict, a love addict, constantly searching for "the one" in hopes that she would bring an end to my troubles and have everything feel right in my universe once more.

Woman after woman, my insatiable addiction grew. I got high just thinking about it; maybe today is the day, maybe the one will stroll into this café, meet my gaze, and we'll stroll out together into the sunset. Maybe that's her over there, she's gorgeous. Oh no, probably that one over there, she's beautiful. No, that one, that one, that one... Even online, each new friend request or follow came with that glimmer of possibility. "No more matches in your area," thumbs throbbing from swiping through dating apps. Two years into my union, the longest unbroken relationship I've ever had, my addiction finally made itself known to me. When it did... everything changed.

There I was, a twenty-nine-year-old adult man living out his dream life. I was in union with "the one," more intimately connected to my life's purpose than ever before, living on a remote tropical island in the middle of the Pacific, driving my dream car, living a prosperous and abundant lifestyle, communing with the land, ocean, plants and animals every single day, most days multiple hours a day. I had great friends, a deeply fulfilling sex life, a beautifully healthy body, and all the time and space in the world to create whatever I wanted. Yet somehow, I found myself still unsatisfied. It felt like something was missing. Whatever that something was, I was certain it was the thing that was going to make me feel satisfied inside.

In my relationship with my beloved, I looked for that something everywhere. I told my beloved we needed more time together, more intimacy, more deep, heartfelt conversations, more love-making, more romance, more time without technology, more, more, more. I was practically driving her mad. I found myself thinking, "Michael, what the fuck? You are literally the luckiest guy on the face of the planet. What's your deal? Why are you making problems where there aren't any? Coming up with petty things to bitch about?" It was subtle, but it was there. This deep, inner dissatisfaction that unconsciously sought to sabotage my life. The thing that's had me keep the back door open on every single one of my romantic relationships. The dead body in the closet. You know, that thing that keeps us from letting ourselves be genuinely happy and fulfilled in life? Here's how it made itself known to me.

Makenzie and I had been cruising along in our relationship, growing and expanding at lightning speed. We were putting in the work, deep diving into our wounds, our conditioning, our imprinting, shadows, and emotional trauma, whatever you want to call those things that beckon you into misery. Every time something would come up, we would turn inwards and face it, even when we had boat loads of resistance and fear. Ego death after ego death our love continuously deepened, as did our intimacy and our connection with one another.

Then my mind started playing tricks on me, and not the "ha-ha, oh that's funny" kind of tricks either. Something inside me kept making me feel like something was missing, an element of our relationship that would quench my inner longing. We certainly knew how to play. We'd joke, act stupid, make funny sounds and movements, act ridiculous in public, talk like children, pretend we were rap stars, dance around the house naked, only to make fun of ourselves and do it all over again. I'm not kidding, the play vibes were real. I loved that about us. It made even the most boring experiences, like driving down the same road to go to the same place for the millionth time, fun.

My mind, however, started making stuff up about it. "We play too much and don't act like serious adults enough. All this childlike behavior is really impacting our intimacy, and not in a good way either. I want more intimacy, more sensuality, more passion, more fire, the kind of tantric love I see everyone posting about these days. Like those photos on Instagram where she's straddling him, arms and legs wrapped around his body, the two lovers clearly on the verge of passionate love-making." Funny how they make you forget there's someone there taking the photo, that it's all staged. It got to the point where I was secretly exploring couple's workshops, as to not offend or hurt my beloved's feelings, anything where we could come together and deepen our experience of intimacy, especially sexually.

Something you ought to know is that this was not the first time I had ever felt this way. This feeling of the infatuation flatlining had surfaced for me in every one of my romantic relationships. Once it settled in, I'd start coming up with what I thought were problems; habits I didn't approve of, behaviors I didn't like, playfulness that I judged as childlike. It would usually go on for so long unexpressed that once I did express it, it came out in a hurtful way, marking the beginning of the end of the relationship. From my perspective, I was always justified in moving on. The women I dated were always confused as to how we could go from being so "in love" to being so broken up in such a short period of time. Hang in there, I promise this is leading somewhere.

Normally when this feeling would surface in my relationships, I would lead with blame. I feel like you ____________ (insert appropriate projection of my feeling onto her behavior). This time was different though. This time my beloved and I both knew something was up with me. This had been going on for far too long now. She, being the incredible woman that she is, had done everything in her power to appease me, sometimes in ways that empowered her and sometimes in ways that disempowered her. She had been extremely patient with me, but the jig was up. After a rather confusing and emotionally triggering conversation, the next day we sat down face to face. It was obvious that it was time for me to part ways with my ego, but I wasn't exactly sure which part. Shortly into our conversation, it all become clear.

Hunger. My body was addicted to being "in love." I had trained it to be. When the infatuation chemicals ran out, I would bail, only to pursue the next relationship/lover/infatuation, starting the cycle all over again. This being the longest relationship I had ever been in, my infatuation chemicals had run out. Up until now, I had related to that as a relationship problem rather than a Michael problem.

My entire adult life I had been caught up in a pattern of beginning relationships with women (be them sexual, romantic, or both) for their promise of fulfillment (sex, love, happiness, etc.), indulging in the "in love" chemicals for as long as they lasted. When the love chemicals ran out, as they always did, I blamed it on my partner. Because of X, Y, and Z, she clearly isn't the one for me. Instead of catching my own pattern, I'd quickly moved on to the next girl and start the cycle back up again.

I was addicted to the newness of things, to the way infatuation felt in my body. I'd let the infatuation consume me, that way it could do its job of distracting me from all the areas of my life that weren't working. Riding one high after the next kept me from having to face my own inner dissatisfaction; the fact that I didn't feel close to my family, that I didn't have my career path figured out, that I hadn't ever experienced being financially independent, that I felt like I was failing at finding my way in the world, that I felt like I could barely support myself, let alone the other person I was dating.

It finally dawned on me. My entire adult life had been run by this shadow of hunger. In my case, it was my hunger for the abstract feminine and her promise of bounty, a lifetime of bliss. Everywhere I went and in everything I did, in the background I was always asking, "are you the one? Are you the one? Are you the one that's going to take away my dissatisfaction and make me all better?" Just so we're clear, I'm not saying that "the one" isn't a real thing. I have found my one and she is the most sacred gift I have ever received. But she didn't save me from my problems. In fact, she pointed them out to me by saying, "hey, you really ought to look at this." It's been my experience that my beloved didn't actually lead me away from my shadow, but instead, led me straight into it. Our relationship brought me face to face with what I had been running from my entire adult life.

I had burned through women like clockwork, drinking in the chemical cocktail of infatuation, getting my fix and getting the hell out. My brain and body were feeding off the high, but my heart was atrophying inside. How was this possible? How could I have missed this rather obvious pattern for so long? It's like any addiction I suppose, evading our awareness until one day we realize it's a problem. My addiction, previously unknown to me, was threatening to sabotage my life, especially my relationship with my beloved. It was having me miss the adventure of what was already right here in front of me. It was having me avoid feeling some really uncomfortable things, things that inevitably led me to deepen my relationship with myself.

I had to have compassion for myself though. Even though I knew my beloved was the woman for me, my physical body was going through withdrawals. I was feeling the effects of the substance shortage, one that every addict must feel once the addictive substance is removed. By design, we're meant to have this hunger. It's a normal part of our hero's journey, what drives us to be successful in whatever ways we define success. When it runs us unconsciously, however, we go our entire lives seeking fulfillment and satisfaction outside of ourselves.

We're on to the next thing without ever letting life fully hit us, letting it really sink in. We leapfrog from woman to woman, getting our fix, never staying long enough to face our shadow. We make problems where there aren't any, project our dissatisfaction, and use all of this as a justification for unconsciously continuing our cycle of addiction. It's a massive blind spot, at least it was for me. Ironically, true love is our only way out. It starts with recognizing how helplessly trapped we are by our hunger and bringing love to that part of us. Love is the key, but what does that even mean?

As our heart opens, we naturally come to the awareness that nothing outside of us can ever fulfill our inner longing for satisfaction; no relationship, career, business success, sexual encounter, money, or material good. We know this conceptually. It's posted about on social media every single day. However, getting it in an embodied way often evades us. When I got how controlled I was by this shadow of hunger, I walked up stairs, took my beloved in my arms, and balled my eyes out. I thanked her for saving my life. Had she not been brave enough to reflect my hunger back to me, I'm certain it would have run the show for the rest of my life.

What was left in the aftermath of such a revelation was a profound sense of freedom and adventure. I felt like I could finally settle in, make myself at home, and get present to the intimacy that had been here in our relationship all along. The feeling of excitement returned, and this time, I don't suspect it will ever go away. I felt relieved, like I had finally passed the test and learned the lesson. The hunger isn't gone. It will likely always be there to some degree or another, but I'm able to be with it rather than be dominated by it. It's something I'm here to work on, reopening my heart to the grand adventure of everyday life. Most of life is filled with monotonous doing. I'm finding that the play I once rejected, ironically, is the exact recipe for experiencing the adventure of the ordinary.

It's no longer my beloved's responsibility to satisfy my hunger. It was never her responsibility to begin with. I no longer have to make problems where there aren't any, and she no longer has to sacrifice her own alignment trying to appease me. It's really a win-win. The energy that was once getting consumed by my unconscious addiction has been liberated to go to work elsewhere, towards my creations, towards my union, and certainly towards delighting in everyday life.

In life we're constantly searching for fulfillment through external means; through sex, substances, romance, and relationships. Even seemingly positive things like the next personal and professional development program, course, or self-help book can have us fall into the trap of thinking, if I do that then I'll finally feel fulfilled and satisfied. If we allow ourselves to contemplate it long enough, our awareness of hunger's presence in our lives will have our bodies start to balance out their internal chemistry once again. Naturally, we'll come more fully into our heart, our one true source of fulfillment and satisfaction. We'll gradually stop seeking and start realizing that fulfillment and satisfaction are an inside job.

Being free from the belief that sex or anything else for that matter will bring us genuine fulfillment and satisfaction will give us the opportunity to start investing our energy into pouring our hearts into our relationships, creations, and service in the world. There is no limit to what we can create when we're not relying on anything in our external environment for fulfillment and satisfaction. Rather than looking for love in all the wrong places, we'll finally be free to pour our love into the world from the right place, from within, from the heart.

Final Words

Thank you for coming along on this journey with me. I'm undoubtedly a different human being on the other side of having conceived, written, and edited this book. Each chapter was a ceremony for me, one that took me deeper into those uncharted territories of my internal being. Grateful doesn't even begin to capture my feelings. Having spent my entire twenties searching for myself, hungry to unravel the man I knew lived inside of me, crossing over into my thirties feels like the celebration of a new age. I feel like I've finally arrived. My thirties are all about service for me. How can I give back all that I've learned, all that I've experienced? How can I pay it forward?

It's both symbolic and perfect to me that this book will be my very first offering. In many ways I already look back on the material and think to myself, "who wrote that?" It feels like I've already changed so much since then. We're growing up so quickly, all of us together. It's almost as if time itself is speeding up. Nevertheless, it has been my honor and delight to sit down daily and bring my contemplations to life with you.

This book was truly a journey, the first of many. Along the way I've gotten to observe and learn a lot of my natural tendencies, like trying to take really big concepts and fit them all into one chapter. Or, wanting to give you everything I know all in one book. Ah surrender, there you are again my old friend. I've also learned a lot about how I create. Where others channel a message in what seems like an instant, I create much more gradually and methodically. There were times when I labored much longer than I should have over choosing the right word for the impact it would make. Surrender again. I've had to let go of my perfectionist tendencies. Most of my life I've spent trying to be perfectly put together. I'm just not, no one is. Perfectly imperfect, as the cliché goes.

My invitation to you as always is to take what feels right to you and leave the rest. No one outside of you will ever be able to guide you in the way that your higher-self can and already does. If I hoped to achieve anything, it was that reading this book brought you closer to yourself, your own truths, and the wisdom that lies at the center of your heart. I cannot even begin to describe to you with words how entirely extraordinary you are. Forged from stardust, a being far more than form itself, you are exceptional, and you came here for some truly amazing things.

I'm grateful to you, for more than just the simple yet extraordinary fact that you made the time to read this book. I'm grateful for all that you are, the time, the work, and the effort you've put in, that you even chose to be here in this world at a time such as this, a world laden with such striking contrast. The fact that you wake up every single day, put on your clothes, and get back to the work you came here to do inspires me. It's always good to remember that what we heal and transform within ourselves, we heal and transform in the world. As within, so without. Thank you for doing your part in healing our world.

It doesn't stop here. This is only the beginning. There are thousands of men and women in our world starving for what you have, what you've learned, what you've embodied. How will you pay it forward? How will you look back and offer your hand to those just beginning their journey? You're needed now. Your embodiment is needed. The world has never been more polarized, darkness and light. Your light is needed more than you realize. Will you be that lighthouse for your brothers and sisters? Will you help them navigate these stormy seas?

I know you will, because I know who you are. I bow to you in your brilliance, your majesty, your virtuosity. Thank you for the work you do each and every day, especially when no one else is watching, to open your heart and invite more love into our world. You are worthy and deserving of every bit of recognition and acknowledgement. Please take a moment now to acknowledge yourself. Never before has there been anyone quite like you. Never will there be again.

Oh, the things we will see. These days, I find myself contemplating the next generation, and what I can do to have them feel safe, nurtured, and encouraged in becoming whomever they're meant to be. Because of the work we're doing, they're entering into the world without any of the same baggage that we had. It's hard to imagine what kind of life experience they'll have, what they'll go on to create, what the world will look like when they become adults and have families of their own. I feel passionate about creating a world worthy of their innocence, and yet I know that it's not entirely up to me. I know I am only one of many men and women committed to creating that kind of world.

How you do sex is how you do life. For all of our sake, and for the sake of those to come, do it with love. Allow love to be the focus of your love-making. Our sacred sexual energy was gifted to us as our means to conceive, nurture, and birth love into the world. You came here to pour forth that love despite your early life conditioning. You were made for that. That is the truest expression of who you really are. Stand in it. Own it. Take your place among the sacred defenders. Protect the innocence, honor the feminine, restore the heart.

We are the generation that bridges the gap between the old way and the new. We do so with love; fierce, relentless, tender, unconditional love. Ultimately, our sacred unions and the containers we create are our playground for practicing. If we can create lasting love and peace in our divine union, then we will do just fine creating that in our world. If we can reclaim the purity of our sacred sexual life force, then we can effectively protect the innocence of future generations. Everything is related to everything else, and the work we do here in transforming our love-making into a vehicle for unconditional love ultimately serves not only us but all of humanity.

Smile. It's not meant to be so hard. The more we can traverse this path with a sense of light-heartedness, the better off we'll be. Trust your body in its healing process and always remember, the body is the last to fully surrender and heal. The most difficult piece of restoring the heart back into our sexuality is often how we treat ourselves when we fail. We will fail at times, that's inevitable. Who will you be for yourself in those moments? Will you still choose love, even when you're the one in need of it? I invite you to be compassionate towards yourself and our human condition. Remember, human AF means equal parts pain and pleasure. Accept both and reap the reward of a truly fulfilling life.

You've got this. This book wouldn't have landed in your lap if that wasn't the case. Trust in yourself, your intuition, and your instincts more than you have at any other point in your life. They are yours for a reason. They chose you.

Restoring the heart into human sexuality is one of the major ways we'll heal the outstanding wounds between men and women, restoring balance between the masculine and the feminine, restoring right relations. As much as our journeys are specifically tailored to us, this is work that men and women must do together. As men, it's time for us to take the lead. No more dragging our feet and making our women suffer trying to get us to grow. It's on us now, it's our responsibility, it's our privilege. When you step onto this path full-heartedly, you'll recognize that for yourself.

Thank you for loving yourself through this process. Thank you for showing up for yourself, for your beloved, for your family, and for the world. And most importantly, thank you for investing your time in making our world a better place for the ones to come. How lucky we are to live such a life. Honoring you immensely for leaning in. Keep going.

About the Author

Michael McPherson is the co-founder of KAKAO Ceremonial Drinking Chocolate, a non-profit devoted to saving native stains of cacao and making ceremonial-grade cacao available to the Western world, and co-founder of KAPU, a community app for light workers to share their heart-centered gifts, services, and wisdom in a safe and sacred space. He's a pioneer in the realm of sacred sexuality, intimacy, inner child work, sacred masculinity, divine union, and heart centered living and leading, with a passion for embodiment, protecting innocence, and restoring right relations between men and women. He's an advocate for Mother Earth and anything linked to preserving, protecting, and regenerating the natural world. Michael lives and works in Maui, Hawaii, with his beloved wife Makenzie.

For more information about Michael, his touring schedule, his future publications, to invite him to speak on a podcast or at an event, or hire his services, please visit his website:

www.michaelmcpherson.co

Acknowledgments

It takes a village to bring a book to life. Never again will I mistake an author as the sole contributor to a creative endeavor like this. Privileged doesn't even begin to describe how I feel about having collaborated with so many inspiring individuals on this project, without whom, you would not be holding this book in your hands.

Thank you to John Hunt and the John Hunt Publishing team for taking a chance on a first time author. Your belief in the success of this endeavor came at a time when I needed it most. Many thanks to all the team members that contributed behind the scenes, whose energy and effort are captured in these pages.

Thank you to Tim Ward, the heartbeat of Changemakers Books, for inspiring a young man to follow his dream. Your challenge to me, to make this material more digestible to my target audience, helped me refine this message for maximal impact. Your communication style, both honest and caring, made collaborating with you all the more satisfying and delightful. Thanks for being a full "fuck yes" to Mak and I, even against your better judgment.

To my editor, Michelle Auerbach, thank you for distilling this material down to the essential. You made the detachment process smooth and seamless, while helping me see its bigger picture application. I thoroughly enjoyed our conversations, seasoned with laughter. Being invited to your dinner table meant the world to me. You're an incredible mother.

Special thanks to my friend Aydin Rahmi for finding the perfect publisher and providing such strong background support throughout the entire book publishing process, and my friend Caitlin Grace for your incredible genius with the cover.

Thank you to my "ride or die" KAPU family for sustaining me through this journey. Your love continually breaks down the barriers around my heart, overflows my cup, and fills me with such faith in humanity. All I want to do is grow old with you, watch our children play together, drink cacao and reminisce about our countless victories over darkness.

To the KAKAO tribe, you were there for the beginning of all this, back when I felt like a wee little baby. Thank you for always supporting me, for sharing the medicine, and for being brave enough to drink it yourselves. Keep igniting this world with your passions. Your medicine is needed now more than ever.

To Gaia, the spirit of Mother Earth, I am eternally indebted to you. Thank you for placing your heart in mine, for brining me back from the dead, for trusting me with this message. I will serve you humbly, always.

Lastly, thank you to my beautiful wife, Makenzie. Who would I be if not for your love? You saw the man in me long before I ever saw him in myself. You, everything that you are, every part of you that you've worked so hard to reclaim, restore, and recover, inspired this work. Thank you for sticking with me, through the good times and the bad, for devoting just as much of your love, energy, and time into this project as I did, for standing for it when I was ready to give up, and for living your life in such a way that made all of this possible. You are by far the most extraordinary human being I've ever met. I'm lucky to call you my wife. I love you, with ALL of my heart, now and always.

Michael McPherson

CHANGEMAKERS
BOOKS

TRANSFORMATION

Transform your life, transform your world - Changemakers Books publishes for individuals committed to transforming their lives and transforming the world. Our readers seek to become positive, powerful agents of change. Changemakers Books inform, inspire, and provide practical wisdom and skills to empower us to write the next chapter of humanity's future. If you have enjoyed this book, why not tell other readers by posting a review on your preferred book site.

Recent bestsellers from Changemakers Books are:

Integration
The Power of Being Co-Active in Work and Life
Ann Betz, Karen Kimsey-House
Integration examines how we came to be polarized in our dealing with self and other, and what we can do to move from an either/ or state to a more effective and fulfilling way of being.
Paperback: 978-1-78279-865-1 ebook: 978-1-78279-866-8

Bleating Hearts
The Hidden World of Animal Suffering
Mark Hawthorne
An investigation of how animals are exploited for entertainment, apparel, research, military weapons, sport, art, religion, food, and more.
Paperback: 978-1-78099-851-0 ebook: 978-1-78099-850-3

Lead Yourself First!
Indispensable Lessons in Business and in Life
Michelle Ray
Are you ready to become the leader of your own life? Apply simple, powerful strategies to take charge of yourself, your career, your destiny.
Paperback: 978-1-78279-703-6 ebook: 978-1-78279-702-9

Burnout to Brilliance
Strategies for Sustainable Success
Jayne Morris
Routinely running on reserves? This book helps you transform your life from burnout to brilliance with strategies for sustainable success.
Paperback: 978-1-78279-439-4 ebook: 978-1-78279-438-7

Goddess Calling

Inspirational Messages & Meditations of Sacred Feminine Liberation Thealogy

Rev. Dr. Karen Tate

A book of messages and meditations using Goddess archetypes and mythologies, aimed at educating and inspiring those with the desire to incorporate a feminine face of God into their spirituality.

Paperback: 978-1-78279-442-4 ebook: 978-1-78279-441-7

The Master Communicator's Handbook

Teresa Erickson, Tim Ward

Discover how to have the most communicative impact in this guide by professional communicators with over 30 years of experience advising leaders of global organizations.

Paperback: 978-1-78535-153-2 ebook: 978-1-78535-154-9

Meditation in the Wild

Buddhism's Origin in the Heart of Nature

Charles S. Fisher Ph.D.

A history of Raw Nature as the Buddha's first teacher, inspiring some followers to retreat there in search of truth.

Paperback: 978-1-78099-692-9 ebook: 978-1-78099-691-2

Ripening Time

Inside Stories for Aging with Grace

Sherry Ruth Anderson

Ripening Time gives us an indispensable guidebook for growing into the deep places of wisdom as we age.

Paperback: 978-1-78099-963-0 ebook: 978-1-78099-962-3

Striking at the Roots
A Practical Guide to Animal Activism
Mark Hawthorne
A manual for successful animal activism from an author with first-hand experience speaking out on behalf of animals.
Paperback: 978-1-84694-091-0 ebook: 978-1-84694-653-0

Readers of ebooks can buy or view any of these bestsellers by clicking on the live link in the title. Most titles are published in paperback and as an ebook. Paperbacks are available in traditional bookshops. Both print and ebook formats are available online.

Find more titles and sign up to our readers' newsletter at
http://www.johnhuntpublishing.com/transformation
Follow us on Facebook at
https://www.facebook.com/Changemakersbooks